Faten LIMAIEM
Nadia BOUJELBENE
Leila BOUHAJJA

Practical Guide to Macroscopy in Pathological Anatomy

Faten LIMAIEM
Nadia BOUJELBENE
Leila BOUHAJJA

Practical Guide to Macroscopy in Pathological Anatomy

Digestive Pathology

ScienciaScripts

Imprint

Any brand names and product names mentioned in this book are subject to trademark, brand or patent protection and are trademarks or registered trademarks of their respective holders. The use of brand names, product names, common names, trade names, product descriptions etc. even without a particular marking in this work is in no way to be construed to mean that such names may be regarded as unrestricted in respect of trademark and brand protection legislation and could thus be used by anyone.

Cover image: www.ingimage.com

This book is a translation from the original published under ISBN 978-3-8416-3779-6.

Publisher:
Sciencia Scripts
is a trademark of
Dodo Books Indian Ocean Ltd. and OmniScriptum S.R.L publishing group

120 High Road, East Finchley, London, N2 9ED, United Kingdom
Str. Armeneasca 28/1, office 1, Chisinau MD-2012, Republic of Moldova, Europe
Printed at: see last page
ISBN: 978-620-0-43854-6

Contents

Foreword

In this book, dedicated to protocols for the macroscopic management of digestive, gynaecological and other surgical specimens, we delve deep into pathological anatomy to explore the detailed and essential intricacies of macroscopy. As pathologists and healthcare professionals, a thorough understanding of the protocols for macroscopic management of surgical specimens is crucial to ensuring accurate diagnoses and optimal patient management.

This comprehensive manual is aimed at practitioners wishing to perfect their macroscopic skills and deepen their expertise in the analysis of operative specimens of digestive origin. By exploring the practical guidelines and techniques specific to each type of operative specimen, this guide aims to provide a comprehensive and detailed resource to support pathologists in their day-to-day practice.

This manual aims to become an indispensable companion, offering clear protocols, relevant illustrations and practical advice for a methodical and rigorous approach to macroscopy in pathological anatomy.

Introduction

At the heart of the practice of pathological anatomy lies the art of macroscopic examination, a crucial stage in the analysis of surgical specimens. Each specimen, meticulously studied, measured, weighed, palpated and dissected, reveals essential clues about the underlying pathology. Guided by precise diagrams and photographs, pathologists embark on a voyage of discovery in which every detail is important.

Macroscopic examination is more than just observation; it guides the prognosis of the disease by identifying key parameters such as lesion size and location, thus guiding choices for subsequent microscopic analysis. From selecting the areas to be sampled to preserving specimens for further investigation, each stage is crucial to ensuring accurate diagnoses.

Fixation, an essential stage, preserves cell morphology and requires particular attention to ensure reliable results. The precautions taken during fixation, such as the choice of the right fixative, the size of the container and specific techniques depending on the nature of the tissue, are all essential links in the specimen processing chain.

Let's delve into the subtleties of impregnation and embedding, the delicate processes that complete the transformation of specimens into paraffin blocks ready for microscopic study. Each step in this meticulous process reveals the commitment of anatomopathologists to unlocking the mysteries of pathology, providing invaluable keys to patient care and medical research.

PART I

Digestive Pathology

MACROSCOPIC EXAMINATION OF APPENDECTOMY SPECIMENS

GENERALITY

Appendectomy, a common surgical procedure, is performed to treat appendicular pathology or prevent complications. All appendices removed undergo anatomopathological examination to diagnose the lesions.

All appendectomy specimens undergo systematic histopathological examination. This is currently standard practice in all hospitals in Tunisia.

Inflammatory pathology of the appendix is far more common than tumour pathology. Preoperative detection of precancerous and tumourous lesions of the appendix remains exceptional, despite the contribution of medical imaging. Only anatomopathological examination provides diagnostic certainty.

ANATOMICAL REMINDER

The vermiform appendage is a flexible tube implanted on the inside of the c®cum, where the three trenia converge. Its position in relation to the crecum varies greatly. Most often, the appendix is latero-crecal.

The appendix is shaped like a more or less flexuous cylindrical tube, with a tapering distal tip and a more or less wide proximal base implanted on the crecum.

The proximal portion is horizontal, attached by the appendicular artery. The distal portion is vertical. The appendicular tip may be connected to the right ovary by adhesions, sometimes forming a true appendiculo-ovarian ligament. The meso-appendix connects the appendix to the ileum and contains the appendicular vessels and nerves.

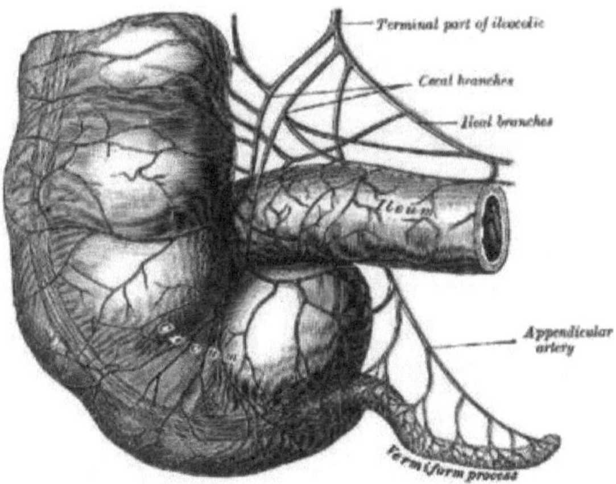

Figure 1: Anatomy of the appendix

Anatomy of the appendix - Department of General and Digestive Surgery, Hopital Saint-Antoine (aphp.fr)

METHODOLOGY

A. Orienting the appendix

4 The first step in the anatomopathological examination of an appendectomy specimen is to **orientate** the operative specimen.

4 The appendix is made up of a **BASE** - a **BODY** - and a **POINT**.

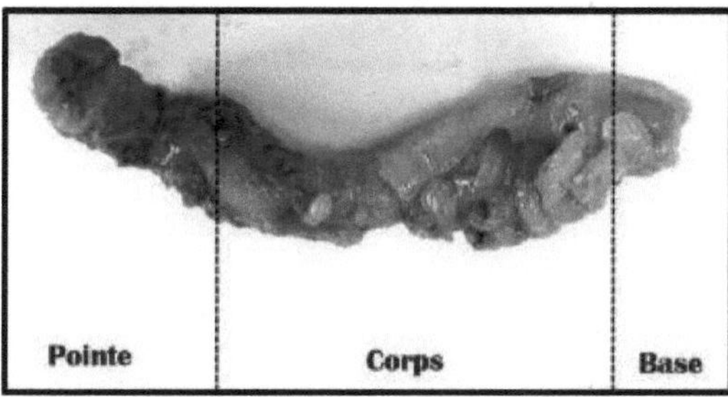

Figure 2: Components of the appendix

Description of the piece and associated lesions:

4 The lump and associated lesions are described: filiform, tumoured, suppurated, perforated with fibrin deposits, dilated or mucocele, diverticulum, etc. Description of the lumen: free, mucus, stercolith, haemorrhage, etc.

Aspect of peritonitis

Colour

Perforation: present / absent

Presence/absence of tumour lesions

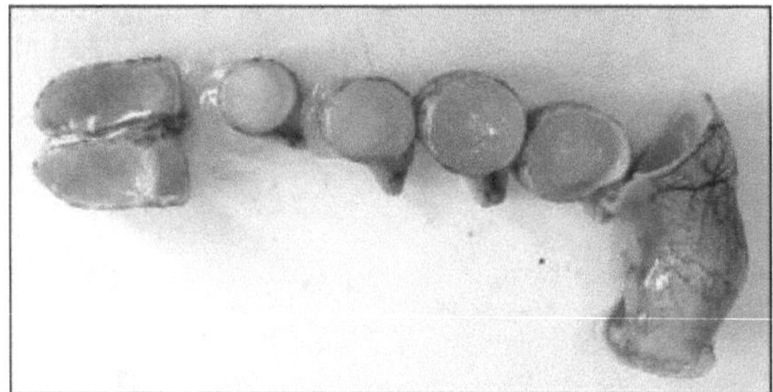

Figure 3: Macroscopic appearance of an appendicular mucocele. The appendicular lumen is distended and filled with abundant mucoid material.

Measure the appendix :

4 Use a flat ruler to measure :

Length: cm

Diameter :   cm

D. Weighing the appendix

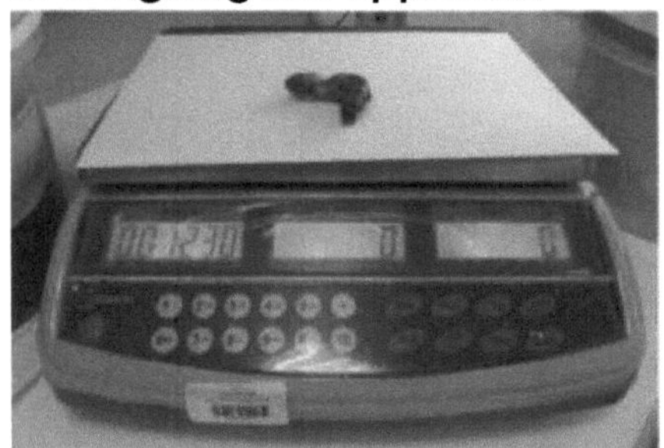

Figure 4 : Weighing the appendix

Isolation of the boundary

4 It can be identified by a notch made with a scalpel.

Macroscopic sections and samples:

Serial cross-sections of the body and description of lesions.

Representative levels of lesions on cassette

Longitudinal section of the tip :

Systematic inclusion of one of the 2 halves (at least)

Description of lesions

Macroscopic Description Sheet :

A specific **macroscopic description sheet** for appendices is desirable, as it provides an exhaustive description that can be included in the pathology report in association with the histological description. The description sheet includes clinical, radiological and macroscopic information on the appendectomy specimens.

6

EXAMEN MACROSCOPIQUE DE L'APPENDICE

■ **Poids** = ...g

■ **Mensurations :**
    → **Longueur** = ...cm
    → **Grand diamètre** = ...cm

■ **Description :**
    → **État :** ....
    → **Aspect Extérieur :** ....
    → **Contenu :**...
    → **Lésion :** ....

■ **Prélèvements :**
    → **Nombre de Fragments**...
    → **Nombre de Cassettes**...

Figure 5: Macroscopic description of appendectomy specimens.

Photographs :

Reproduced appendices may be photographed for the purpose of documenting the case. Photographs may or may not be included in the final report.

MATERIAL REQUIRED

Fixing agent: The usual fixing agent is 10% buffered formalin.
Scalpel blade
Regie plate
Cassettes
Camera

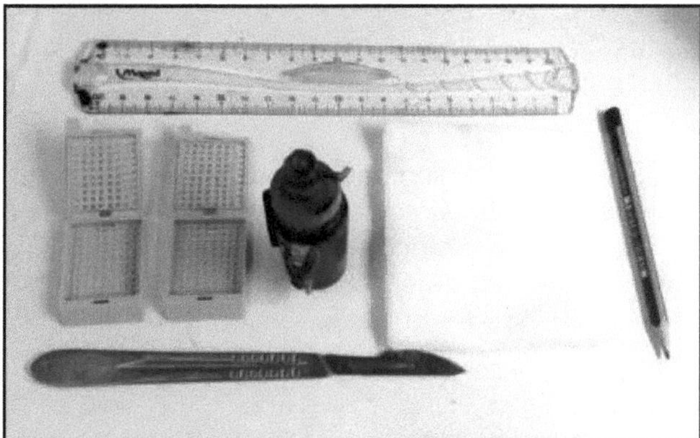

Figure 6: Equipment required for the macroscopic management of gastrointestinal

polyps.

CONDITIONS AND RULES OF GOOD PRACTICE

Appendages are fixed in 10% buffered formalin.

Delayed or poor fixation can alter the morphological quality of histological sections. It is important to respect the ratio of tissue volume to fixative volume (1/10).

All appendices must be sent to the pathology laboratory together with a **clinical information sheet**. This form should include the history of the disease, the patient's antecedents, the results of the paraclinical examinations carried out and the endoscopic data.

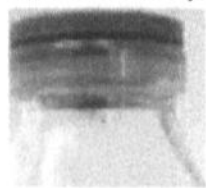

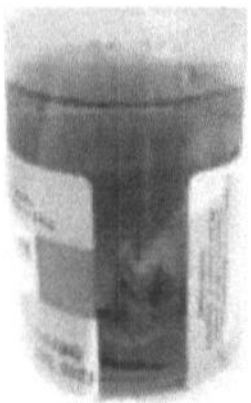

Figure 7: Appendectomy specimen arriving fixed in 10% buffered formalin in a labelled
vial

What to describe?

Appendix dimensions: length, diameter

Description of appendix: filiform, tumoured, suppurated, perforated with fibrin deposits, dilated or mucocele, diverticulum...

Description of the light: free, mucus, stercolith, hemorrhage...

Tumour lesion: location, aspects, dimensions.

What to deduct

Systematic sampling: **base, upper levels** and **tip** (minimum 1 half)

Samples **and** any associated **lesions**

CONCLUSION

Systematic anatomopathological examination of appendectomy specimens reveals a variety of tumourous and non-tumourous lesions requiring further investigation and appropriate therapeutic management.

Macroscopic examination alone cannot detect such lesions, which may go unnoticed. It is therefore recommended that all appendectomies undergo systematic histopathological examination.

I. REFERENCES

Pariente A, Bonnefoy O. Diseases of the appendix. Encycl Med Chir(Elsevier Masson,

Paris), Traite de Medecine Akos, 4-0565, 2013, 5p.

Scoazec JY. Pathology of the appendix. Ann Pathol. 2010;30(2):94-5.

Charfi S, Sellami A, Affes A, YaTch K, Mzali R, Sellami-Boudawara T. Histopathological findings in appendectomy specimens: a study of 24,697 cases. Int J Colorectal Dis. 2014;29(8):1009-12.

Ben Hamed Y. Interet de l'examen anatomo-pathologique systematique de tout appendice ayant subi une ablation chirurgicale [These]. Medecine: Tunis; 1980. 54p.

PART II

TECHNICAL SHEET: MACROSCOPIC EXAMINATION OF A CHOLECYSTECTOMY SPECIMEN

ANATOMY OF THE GALLBLADDER - GENERAL INFORMATION

The normal gallbladder is a small, pyriform sac measuring between 7 and 10 cm in length and around 3 cm in body diameter, depending on how full it is.

It can contain from 40 to 70 ml of bile.

The wall itself is **thin**, measuring **1** to **3 mm**, depending on its state of contraction or relaxation, but it can be thickened by fat around its edges.

On imaging, vesicular parietal thickening occurs when the wall exceeds **5 mm.**

We describe **3** main **parts of** the gallbladder that merit sampling for microscopic analysis.

A distal, blind part, the **vesicular fundus.**

A main part, or **body.**

A narrow proximal part, the **collar** or **vesicular neck**, 5 to 8 mm long

The infundibulum refers to the funnel-shaped area between the body and the collar.

The **vesicular neck** connects to the **cystic duct**, which can be between 2 and 3 cm long.

The lumen of the neck and its junction with the **cystic duct** is incompletely divided by spiral diaphragms which form **Heister's spiral valve.** A lymph node is often attached to the neck.

The gallbladder is surrounded by a **peritoneal sheet** (visceral peritoneum) over 2/3 of its surface, outside the zone of adhesion to the liver parenchyma.

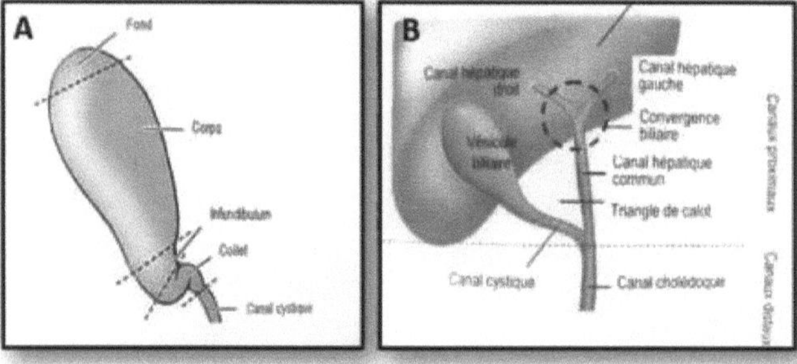

Figures 1A and 1B: Anatomy of the gallbladder

(Reference : Le Bail.B et al. Ann Pathol 2014; 34:258-265)

METHODOLOGY

Orientation :

The narrow funnel-shaped **neck** looks inwards and upwards. There is a light at the end.

Clips are often placed over the **cystic artery** and the **cystic ductal limit.**

The non-peritonealised surface of the gallbladder corresponds to its upper part, adjacent to the liver.

The **vesicular fundus** is large, bulbous and blind; it is directed forwards and outwards.

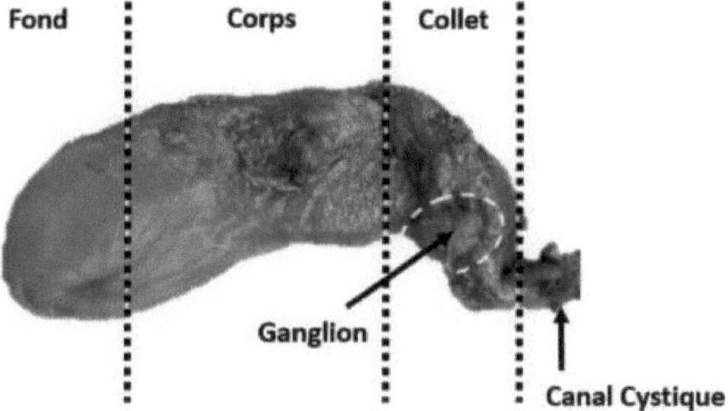

Figure 2: orientation of the gallbladder

Orient the gallbladder and identify any **other structures** removed en bloc: liver (segments IV and/or V most often), bile ducts.

Weighing the cholecystectomy specimen:

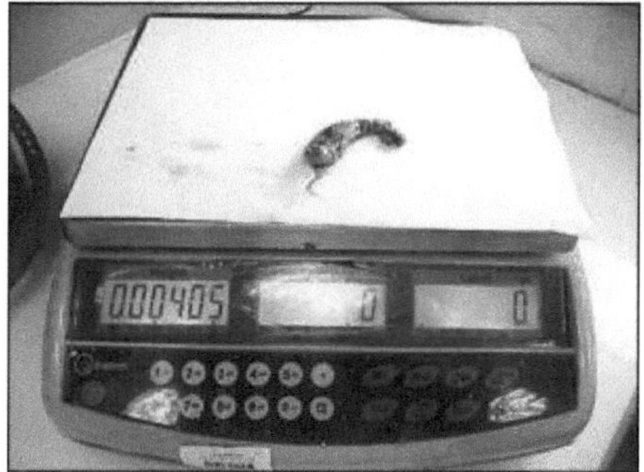

Figure 3: Weighing the cholecystectomy specimen

Measuring the gallbladder
The length
The largest diameter

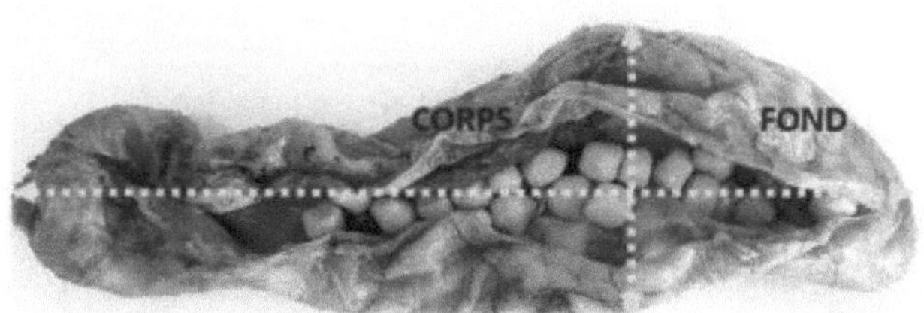

Figure 4: Gallbladder measurements: length and largest diameter

11

Measuring adjacent structures
Length of cystic duct
Neck ganglion
Hepatic fragment and other bile duct segments, if present.
Describe the condition of the gallbladder (open, closed, fragmented, etc.) and its **external appearance** (inflammation, perforation, adhesions).
Collection :
+ Levy
The limit of the cystic duct in cross-section)
The neck ganglion, if identified.
Open the vesicular **sac longitudinally** (with blunt-tipped scissors or a scissor).

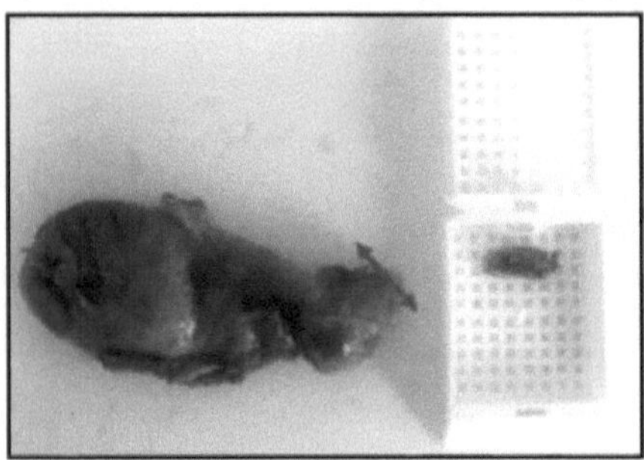

Figure 5: Removal of the vesicular neck

7. carefully, using a scalpel), from the bottom towards the cystic duct.
Empty its contents (bile, pus, lithiasis, etc.) and describe it.

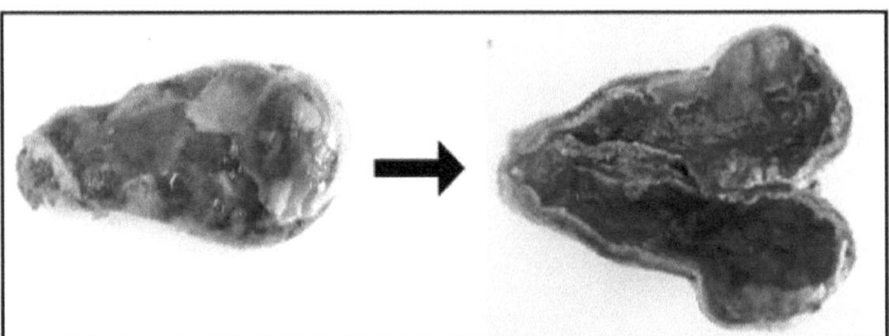

Figure 6: Longitudinal opening of the gallbladder

NB: the bile must be emptied and the mucosa wiped as soon as possible after receipt to avoid corrosion.
Inspect the mucosal surface and **describe** any inflammatory or tumour-like abnormalities.
Slice the entire gallbladder, in transverse slices **3-4 mm** apart.

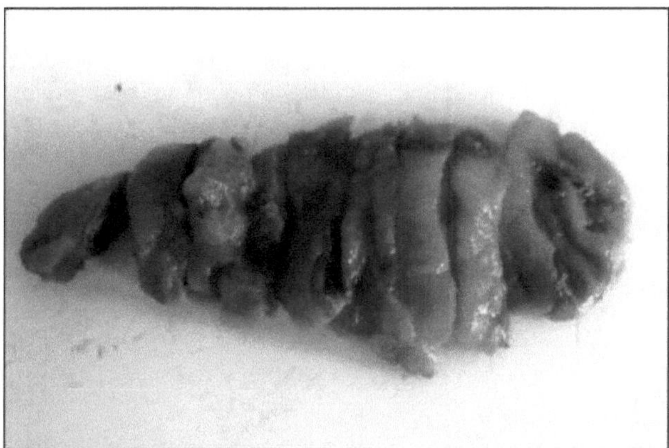

Figure 7: Slicing the entire vesicle, in transverse slices spaced 3-4 mm apart.

Select the fragments of interest and put them in cassettes:
In the absence of macroscopic abnormalities: systematic sampling of the **body** and **fundus**, the whole of which can generally be accommodated **in a single cassette**, together with the **neck** and **lymph node.**

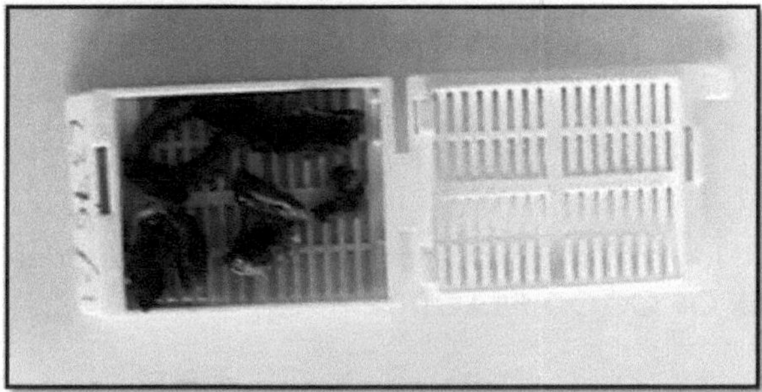

Figure 8: Samples taken from the gall bladder are placed in a cassette.

In the case of macroscopic abnormalities: sample the **lesion** widely on several sections perpendicular to the mucosal surface, taking care to include the **serosal margin.**
In the case of radical resection for vesicular cancer: take a large sample to analyse the relationship of the tumour with the **liver** and **bile ducts**, and sample the **hepatic and biliary borders**; take all the **regional lymph nodes.**
RECAP: WHAT TO TAKE
4 The **cystic border**: circumferential cross-section (systematic).
The **neck node** if identified, and any other nodes that may be communicated individually.
A **partial slice of the body and bottom**, if the macroscopic appearance is normal/subnormal.
All **focal or diffuse lesions**, whether suspected of malignancy or not (ulcerations, perforations, polyps, parietal thickening, etc.): multiple transverse sections, taking

care to visualise the serous border.

4- In the case of **radical resection for vesicular cancer**: the liver and communicated bile ducts (taking care to visualise their relationship with the tumour), the boundaries of these organs, and all regional lymph nodes.

4 If **dysplasia or carcinoma** is found incidentally on microscopic examination, include all macroscopic section slices *retrospectively*.

-I- Vesicular lithiasis will not be sampled.

MATERIAL REQUIRED

1. **Fixing agent:** The usual fixing agent is 10% buffered formalin.
2. **Scalpel blade - knife**
3. **Scissors**
4. **Tape measure - Regie plate**
5. **Cassettes**
6. **Camera**

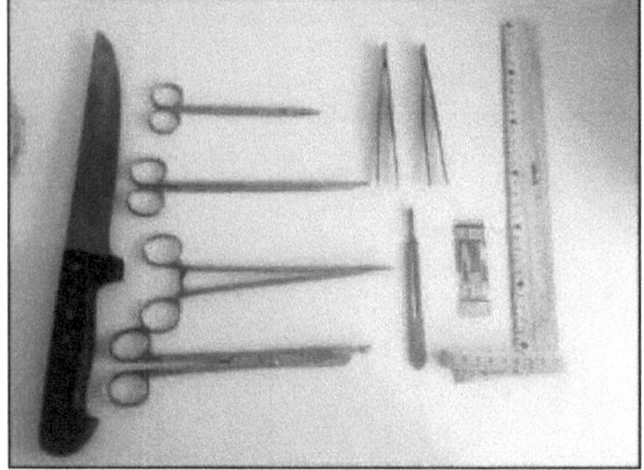

Figure 9: Equipment required for macroscopic examination of the gallbladder

CONDITIONS AND RULES OF GOOD PRACTICE

The surgical specimen is fixed for 24 hours in 10% buffered formalin.

Delayed or poor fixation will impair the morphological quality of histological sections. Respect the ratio of tissue volume to fixative volume (1/10).

All cholecystectomy specimens must be sent to the pathological anatomy laboratory together with a clinical information sheet describing the history of the disease, the patient's antecedents, the results of the practical paraclinical examinations and the treatment instituted.

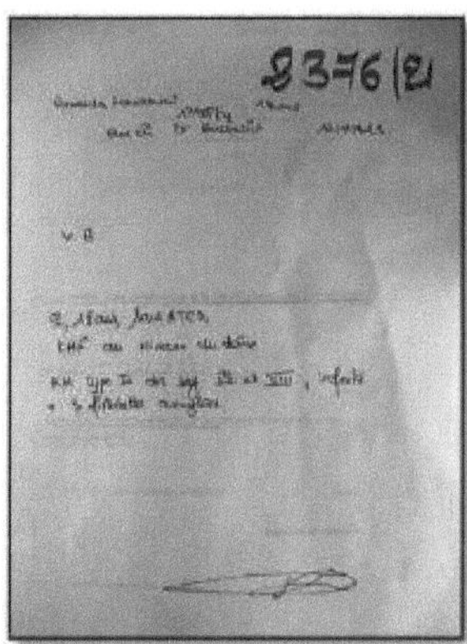

Figure 10: Request form for anatomopathological examination
of a cholecystectomy specimen

CONCLUSION

Systematic anatomopathological examination of cholecystectomy specimens is used not only to confirm or refute the diagnosis of acute or chronic cholecystitis suspected by the clinician, but also to detect various benign, precancerous or malignant lesions, most often of incidental origin, which require further investigation, extension and appropriate therapeutic management.

REFERENCES

S Prevot. Pathology of the gallbladder. Ann Pathol 2014; 34, 279-287.
Couvelard VB pancreas L3 HGE 2014 - Moodle Sorbonne (studylibfr.com).
The Lease. B. Pathology of the gallbladder. Ann Pathol 2014; 34: 258-265.

PART III

MACROSCOPIC EXAMINATION OF DIGESTIVE POLYPS

GENERAL

Colorectal polyps are macroscopic, well-circumscribed, localised lesions protruding into the digestive tract. They may be sessile or pedunculated, of variable size, single or multiple, epithelial or non-epithelial in origin.

This is a macroscopic term which does not prejudge the histological nature of the lesion.

Polypectomies are diagnostic and therapeutic resection procedures. They are being performed more frequently as a result of organised colorectal cancer screening and improvements in interventional endoscopic techniques.

The management of a colorectal polyp depends on a rigorous anatomopathological examination.

ANATOMICAL REMINDER

Pedicle polyps: attached to the mucosa by an elongated foot that is longer than it is wide (**Figure 1**).

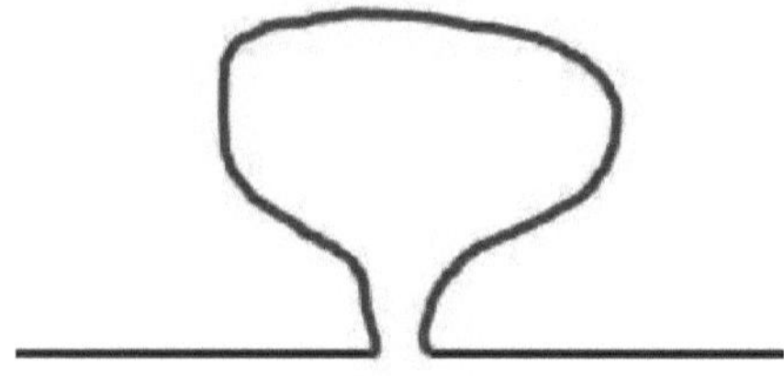

Figure 1: Schematic representation of a pedicle polyp.

Sessile polyps: etales with a wide implantation base (**Figure 2**).

Figure 2: Schematic representation of a sessile polyp

METHODOLOGY

A- Description of the polyp :

Colour :

Shape: Sureleve   PlatExcave

Surface : Smooth   Nodular Villiform   Granular

Configuration (insertion base) : Sessile Pedicle

Ulceration: Present   Absent

Orienting the polyp

The polypectomy specimens must be orientated before cutting, to determine their various constituent parts.

Pedicle polyps: consist of a head, a pedicle and an insertion base (Figure 3).
Sessile polyps: consist of a head and a broad insertion base.

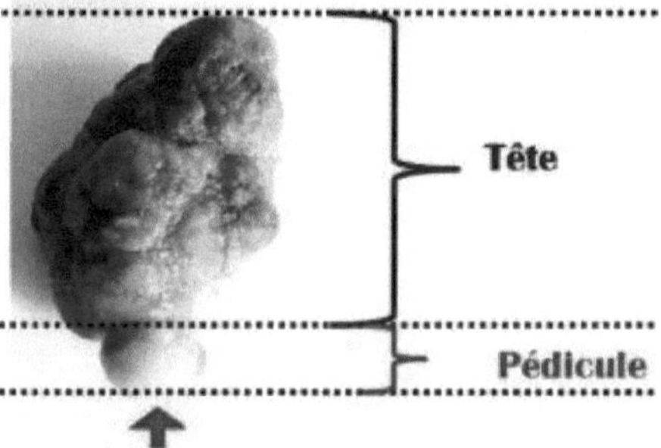

Insertion base

Figure 3: The different components of a pedicle polyp.

C. Measuring the polyp :

A flat ruler is used to measure the different structures of the polyp (**Figure 4**).
∧ Polyp diameter
∧ Pedicle length if present
∧ Diameter of polyp insertion base.

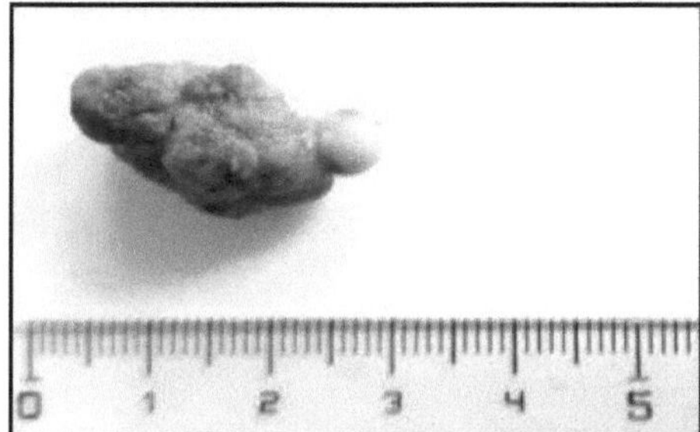

Figure 4: Measurement of the pedicle polyp using a flat ruler.

Inking: the base of the polyp insertion **is inked** with Indian ink (**Figure 5**). Inking is in fact optional because the resection limits are often quite easily identifiable under the microscope by the tissue changes induced by cauterisation.

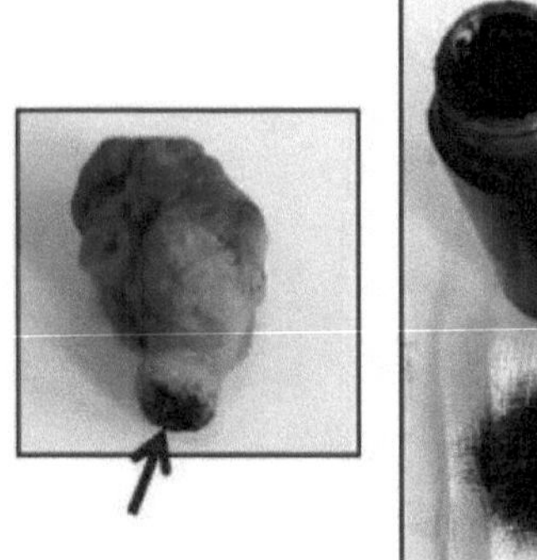
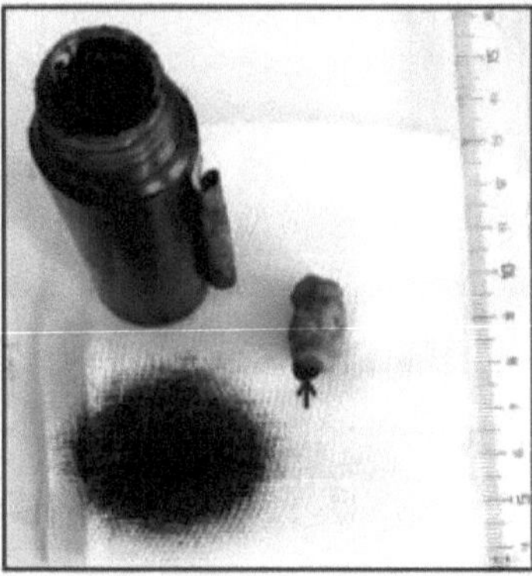

Figure 5: Inking the polyp insertion base with Indian ink.

Macroscopic sections (Figure 6)
Sessile polyps :

<5 mm: included in their entirety as they are without any cutting. En bloc inclusion is performed along the sagittal axis of the pedicle and the polyp is serially cut.

>5mm: serial slices at 3-4mm intervals

Polyps Pedicles

<10mm in diameter: cut through the pedicel

>10 mm in diameter: dissect each side of the pedicle and cut the rest at intervals of 3 to 4 mm.

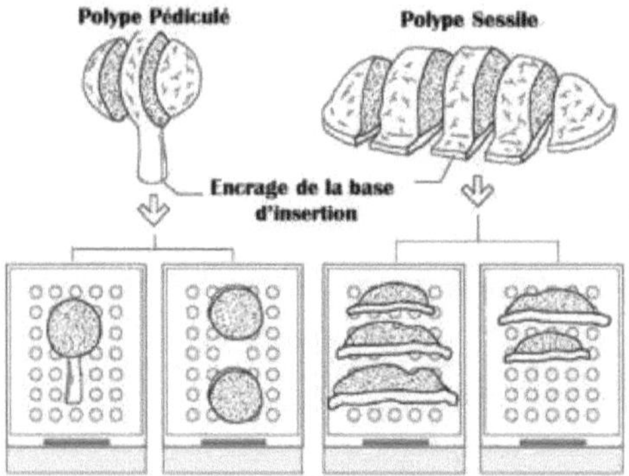

Figure 6: Protocol for macroscopic management of sessile polyps and pedicles https://www.rcpa.edu.au/Manuals/Macroscopic-Cut-Up-Manual/Gastrointestinal/Colorectal/Colorectal-polyp

Placing fragments in cassettes: it is essential to include the whole polyp.

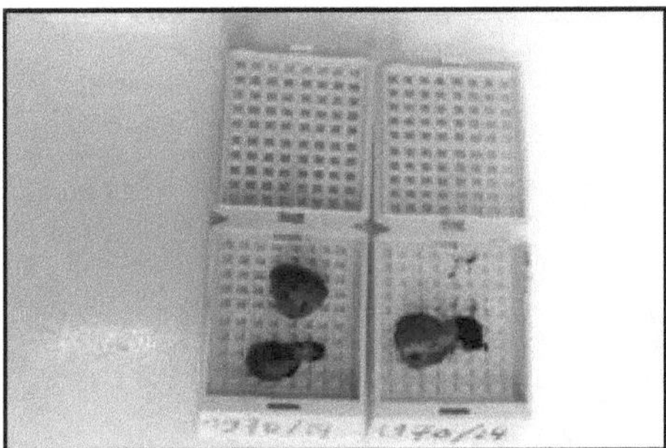

Figure 7: The dissected polyp is placed in two cassettes and fully included.

Macroscopic Description Sheet :

A specific **macroscopic description form** for digestive polyps **(Figure 8)** is desirable, as it provides an exhaustive description that can be incorporated into the pathology report in association with the histological description. The description form includes clinical, endoscopic and macroscopic information on the polypectomy specimens.

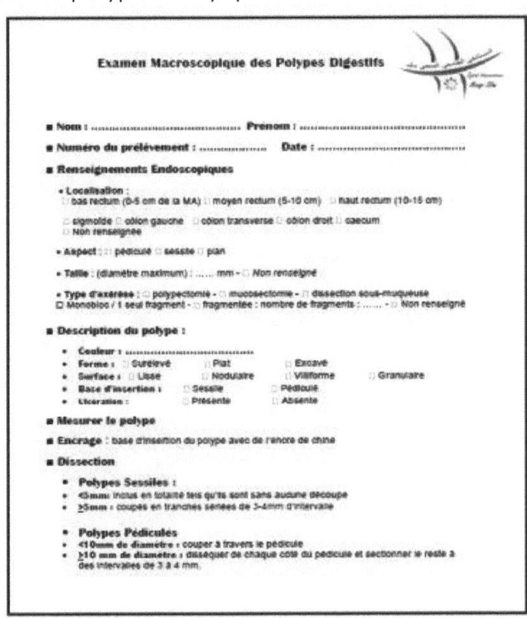

Figure 8: Macroscopic description of digestive polyps.

G. Photographs :

Any polyps found may be photographed for the purposes of documenting the case. Photographs may or may not be included in the final report.

EQUIPMENT REQUIRED (Figure 9)

19

Fixing agent: The usual fixing agent is 10% buffered formalin.
Indian ink
Scalpel blade
Regie plate
Cassettes
Camera

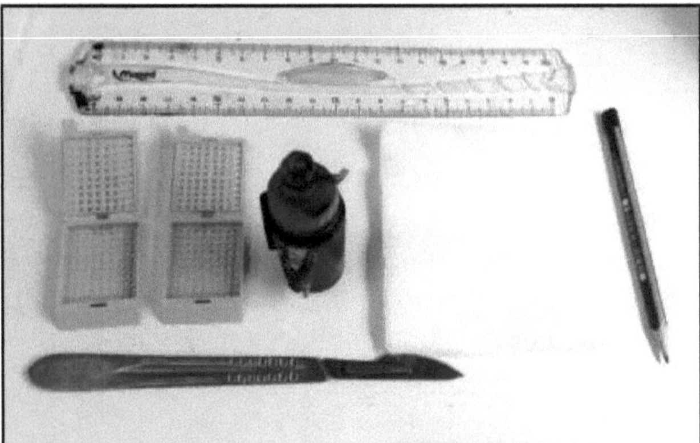

Figure 9: Equipment required for the macroscopic management of gastrointestinal polyps.

CONDITIONS AND RULES OF GOOD PRACTICE

Digestive polyps are fixed in 10% buffered formalin.

Delayed or poor fixation can alter the morphological quality of histological sections. It is important to respect the ratio of tissue volume to fixative volume (1/10).

All digestive polyps must be sent to the pathology laboratory with a **clinical information form (Figure 9)**. This form should include the history of the disease, the patient's antecedents, the results of the paraclinical examinations carried out and the endoscopic data.

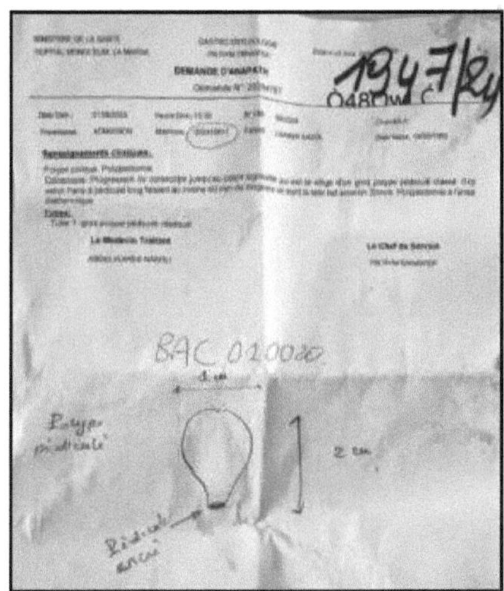

Figure 10: Clinical information sheet accompanying the polypectomy piece

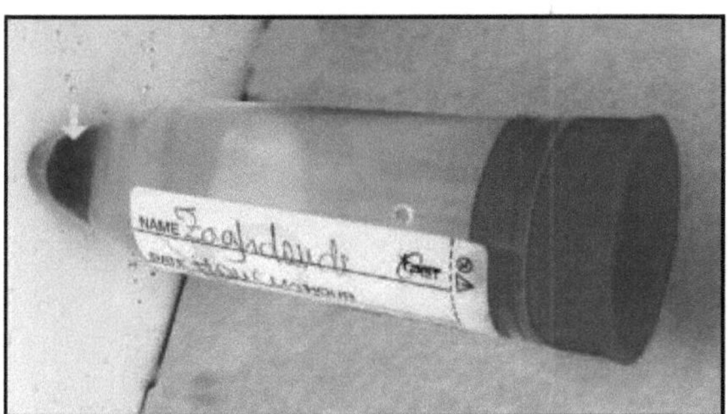

Figure 11: Polypectomy specimen (arrow) in a labelled vial, fixed with 10% buffered formalin

CONCLUSION

- In conclusion, the macroscopic management of digestive polyps plays a crucial role in the accurate assessment of histological features.

By using specialised tools and making thin sections, it is possible to examine specimens in detail, enabling a precise assessment of the degree of dysplasia and the detection of any possible cancerous progression.

This approach, based on appropriate management, contributes to better-informed therapeutic decisions and improved clinical outcomes.

REFERENCES

https://www.pathologyoutlines.com/topic/colontumorfeaturestoreport.html
https://fr.slideshare.net/slideshow/grossing-of-colorectal-specimens/75397463
https://www.rcpa.edu.au/Manuals/Macroscopic-Cut-Up-Manual/Gastrointestinal/Colorectal/Colorectal-polyp

Manual of Surgical Pathology 3rd Edition by <u>Susan C. Lester MD PhD</u>
Brown I, Bourke M, Ackland S, Eckstein R, Hawkins N, Hicks S, Hunter A, Kneebone A, Ruszkiewicz A and Yeong ML. *Polypectomy and local resections of the colorectum structured reporting protocol*, The Royal College of Pathologists of Australasia, Surry Hills, NSW, 2013.

PART IV

MACROSCOPIC MANAGEMENT OF A NON-TUMOUROUS GRAFTED INTESTINAL RESECTION SPECIMEN ANATOMY OF THE SMALL INTESTINE

Small intestine:

Proximal segment of the intestine

Small calibre decreasing from 4 to 2 cm from proximal to distal end

Function: mainly responsible for digestion and absorption of food.

Different segments (proximal - distal) :

Duodenum (20-25 cm)

Jejunum (2.4 m)

Ileum (3.6 m)

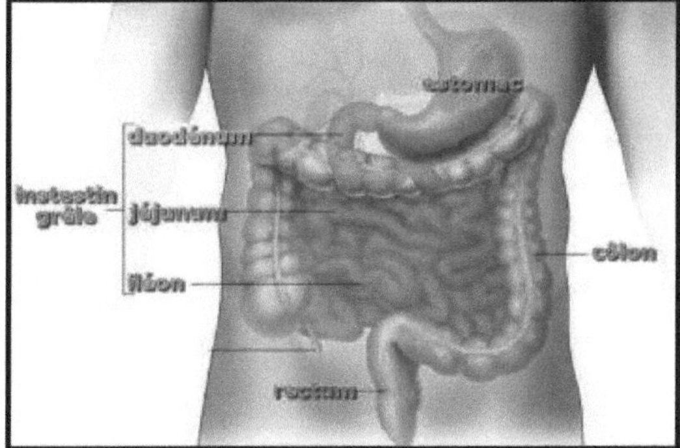

Figure 1: Anatomy of the large intestine
Large intestine: definition and explanations (aquaportail.com)

Guiding criteria :

The duodenum is orientated by the head of the pancreas, which is often associated with the duodenum and which it frames from the outside.

In the case of ileocolic resection, the ileum is oriented via the c^cum, Bauhin's valve and even the appendix if present.

In the case of other segmental resection, if the surgeon fails to identify the extremities beforehand, the segment cannot be oriented.

METHODOLOGY

A- Description of the piece :

0 Specimen **measurement**

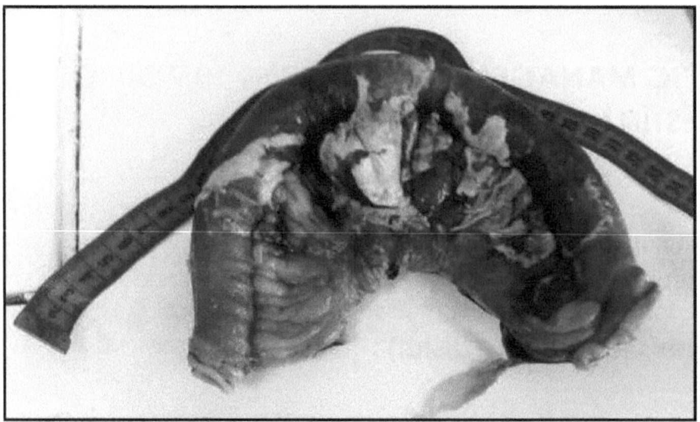

Figure 2 : Measuring the intestinal resection section using a tape measure

0 **Weighing the workpiece**

0 **Description of** the specimen :

Main lesions and

Associated lesions (polyp, appendix...)

Caution: whatever the indication, a search must always be made for an associated tumour lesion.

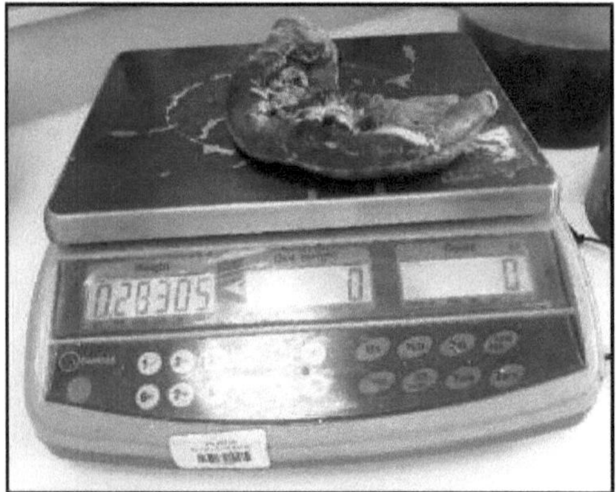

Figure 3: Weighing the piece of grafted intestinal resection

B- Limit sampling :

Longitudinal limits :

After fixation (24-48 hours), the longitudinal edges are removed separately.

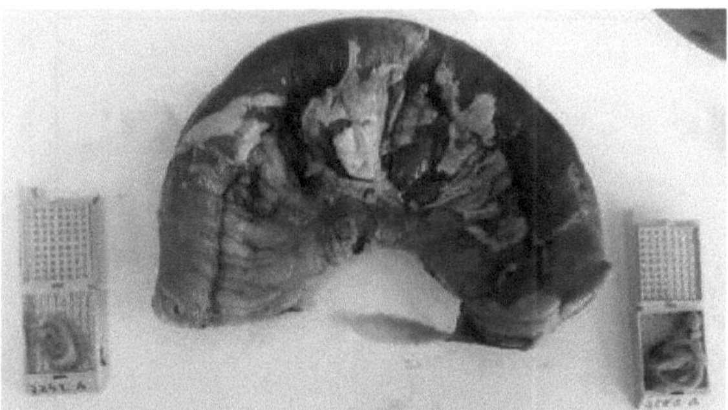

Figure 4: Removal of the two longitudinal surgical resection limits

Proximal vascular pedicle (root of mesentery)

Remove the root of the mesentery and several sections of the vascular pedicle in cases of suspected ischemic lesion

C- Selection of samples :

Cross-section of the entire specimen in **macroscopically serrated slices** in order to identify and remove the lesions most relevant to the diagnosis. Specify their relationship (distance) to the **limits of the exeresis**.

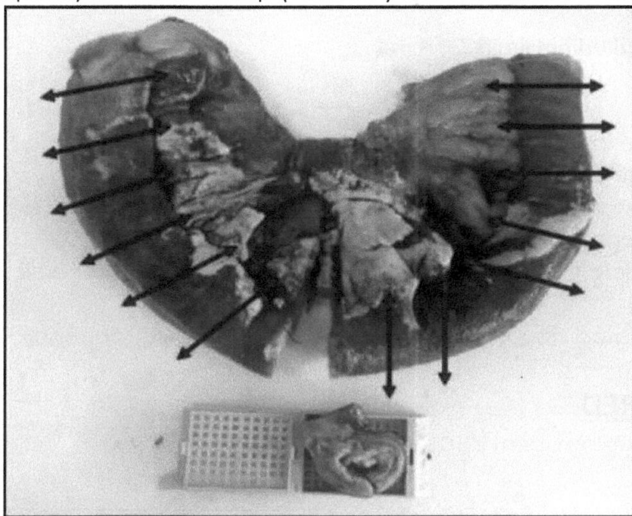

Figure 5: Macroscopically serialised slices and removal of the most relevant lesions

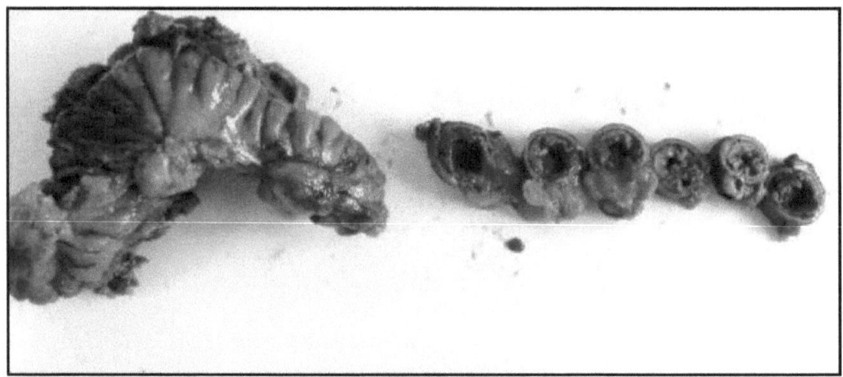

Figure 6: Macroscopically serial slicing of an ileocaecal resection for Crohn's disease

D- Ganglion sampling :

1 or more lymph nodes per cassette without exhaustive search in the absence of associated tumour lesions.

WHAT TO TAKE?

Proximal and distal **longitudinal limits**

Main lesions :

Sampling of the different representative aspects of the lesion

Samples taken at the lesion/healthy wall junction

Systematic sampling of non-lesional walls

Nodes: 1 or more gg/cassette without exhaustive search in the absence of associated tumour lesion.

Proximal vascular pedicle (root of mesentery) in case of suspected ischemic cause

Other lesions or associated tissues: polyps, ulcerations, diverticula, appendix, etc.

MATERIAL REQUIRED

Fixing agent: The usual fixing agent is 10% buffered formalin.

Scalpel blade - knife

Scissors

Tape measure - Regie plate

Cassettes

Camera

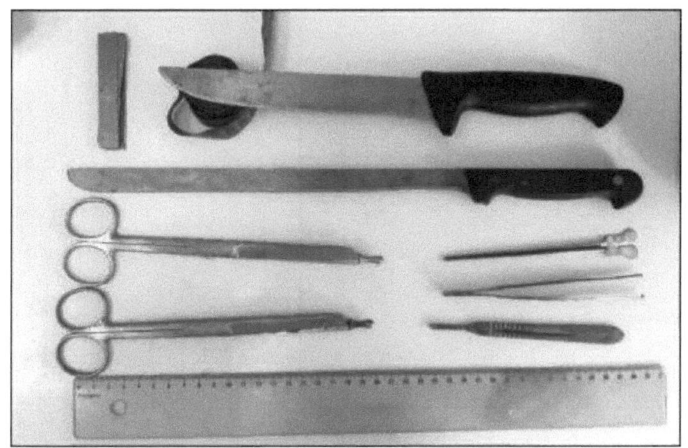

Figure 7: Equipment required for macroscopic processing of intestinal resection specimens

Example 1:

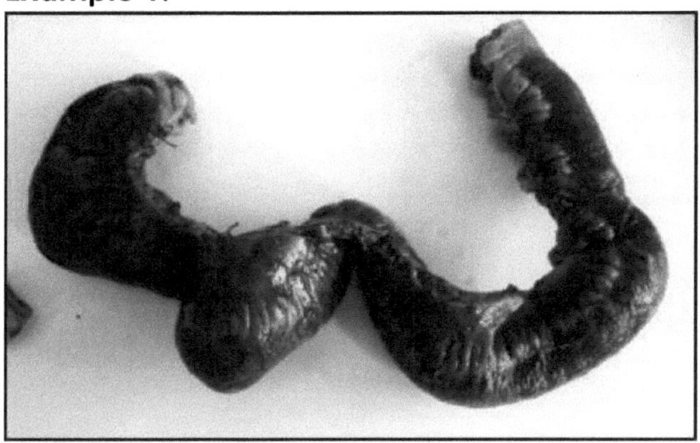

Figure 8: Ischemic necrosis of the small intestine.

Example 2:

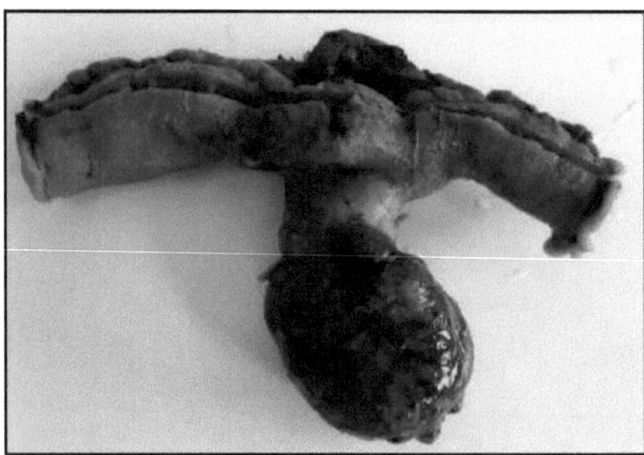

Figure 9: Meckel diverticulum

CONDITIONS AND RULES OF GOOD PRACTICE

The surgical specimen is fixed for 24 - 48 hours in 10% buffered formalin.

Delayed or poor fixation will impair the morphological quality of histological sections. Respect the ratio of tissue volume to fixative volume (1/10).

All intestinal resection specimens must be sent to the pathological anatomy laboratory together with a clinical information sheet detailing the history of the disease, the patient's past history, the results of practical paraclinical examinations and the treatment being administered.

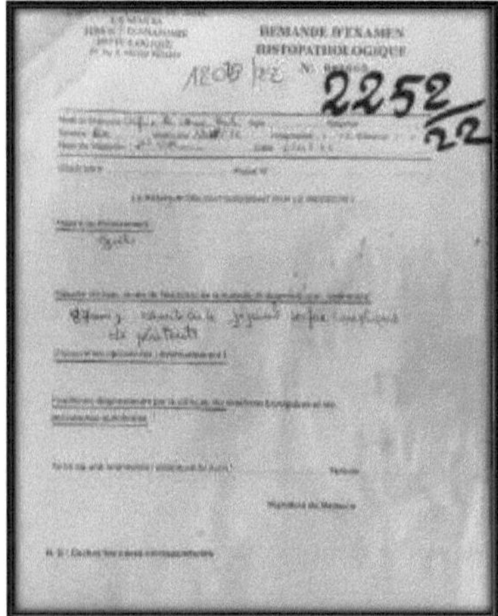

Figure 10: Clinical information sheet accompanying the piece of gallbladder bowel resection received by the pathology laboratory

CONCLUSION

■ Macroscopic examination of grafted intestinal resection specimens contributes to patient management by assessing prognosis and defining important criteria for prescribing any additional postoperative treatment.

REFERENCES

1. DIGESTIVE TUBE.pdf (uca.ma)
2. productfile 2047.pdf (facmed-univ-oran.dz)

PART V

MACROSCOPIC MANAGEMENT OF A TUMOUR GRAFTED INTESTINAL RESECTION SPECIMEN ANATOMY OF THE SMALL INTESTINE

Small intestine:

Proximal segment of the intestine
Small calibre decreasing from 4 to 2 cm from proximal to distal end
Function: mainly responsible for digestion and absorption of food.

Different segments (proximal - distal) :

Duodenum (20-25 cm)
Jejunum (2.4 m)
Ileum (3.6 m)

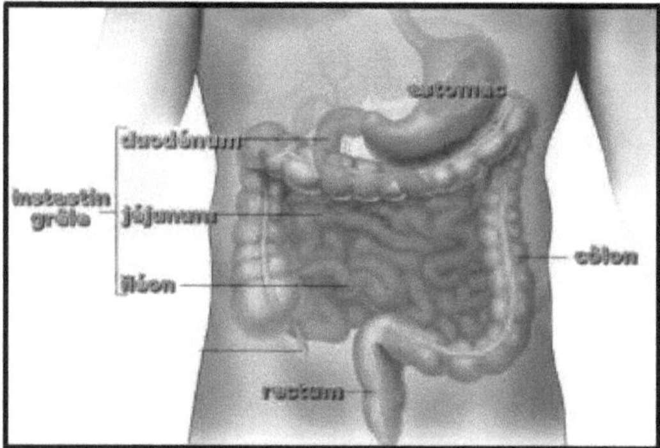

Figure 1: Anatomy of the large intestine
Large intestine: definition and explanations (aquaportail.com)

D. Guiding criteria :

The duodenum is orientated by the head of the pancreas, which is often associated with the duodenum and is surrounded by it from the outside.
In the case of ileocolic resection, the ileum is oriented via the c^cum, Bauhin's valve and even the appendix if present.
In the case of other segmental resection, if the surgeon fails to identify the extremities beforehand, the segment cannot be oriented.

METHODOLOGY

Description and samples of the piece :

Description :

Length of specimen
Weighing the workpiece

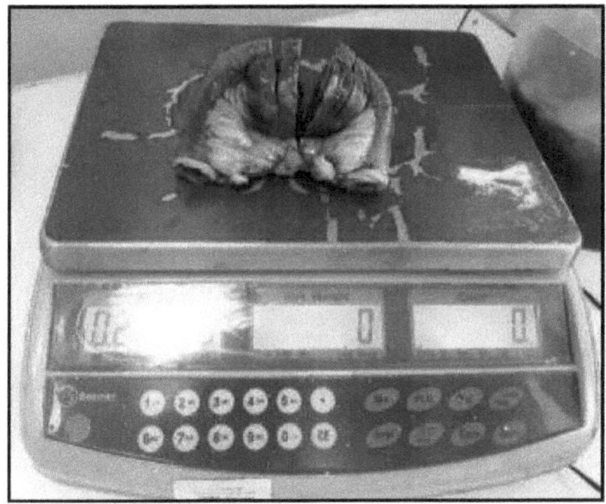
Figure 2: Weight of the tumour-grafted intestinal resection specimen

Main lesion: Appearance, size, relationship to boundaries
Associated lesions
All this information can be summarised on the **macroscopic sheet.**

Collection:

Longitudinal limits: to be taken separately
Tumour: Macroscopically serial sections of the tumour and adjacent meso in order to select the most representative section levels of the tumour, particularly **in areas of maximum infiltration** (3 to 5 levels in the tumour zone), tumour/non-tumour junction.

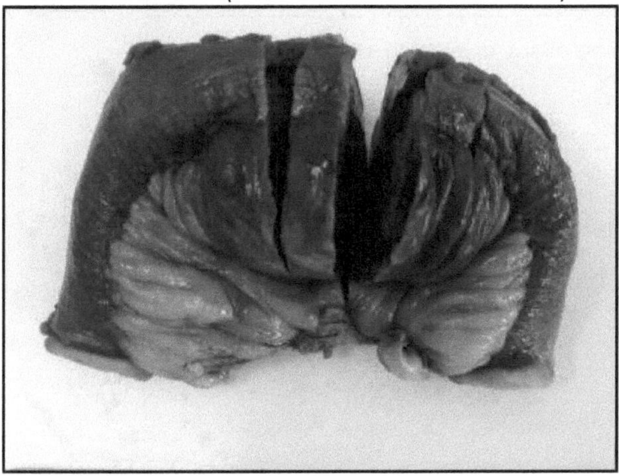
Figure 3: Macroscopically serial sections of the tumour

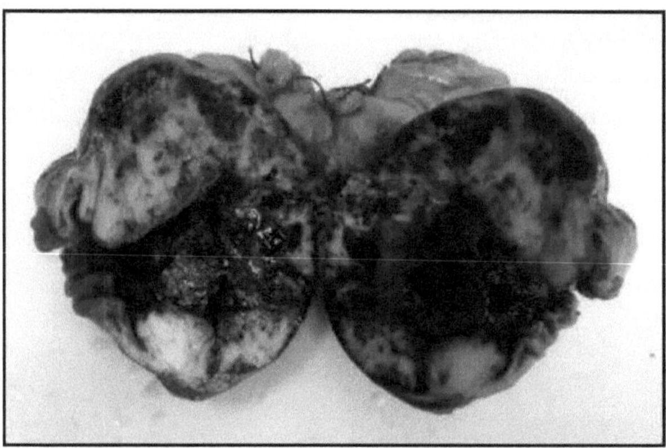

Figure 4: Following macroscopic sections of the tumour, its appearance is described: in this case, the tumour is whitish with sub-mucosal development and is the site of significant hemorrhagic changes.

Peri-tumour nodes: 1 node/cassette and 1 tumour nodule/cassette

Associated lesions.

What to collect

Proximal and distal **longitudinal limits**

Main tumour: maximum tumour infiltration levels and tumour/non-tumour junction (i.e. **3** to **5** slice levels)

Nodes: meticulous search for all nodes, inclusion of all if macroscopically non-tumourous or of part if tumourous, 1gg/cassette. If less than 12 or 8 lymph nodes, repeat the section with or without the aid of complementary techniques.

Associated lesions: polyps, ulcerations, diverticula, appendix, etc.

MATERIAL REQUIRED

Fixing agent: The usual fixing agent is 10% buffered formalin.

Scalpel blade - knife

Scissors

Tape measure - Regie plate

Cassettes

Camera

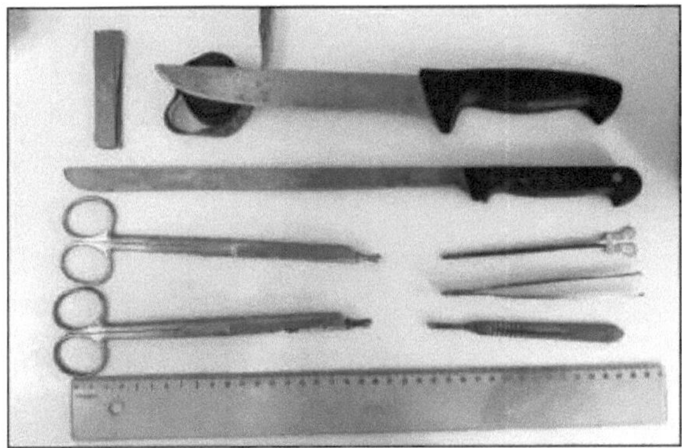

Figure 5: Equipment required for macroscopic processing of intestinal resection specimens

CONDITIONS AND RULES OF GOOD PRACTICE

The surgical specimen is fixed for 24 - 48 hours in 10% buffered formalin.

Delayed or poor fixation will impair the morphological quality of histological sections. Respect the ratio of tissue volume to fixative volume (1/10).

All intestinal resection specimens must be sent to the pathological anatomy laboratory together with a clinical information sheet detailing the history of the disease, the patient's past history, the results of practical paraclinical examinations and the treatment being administered.

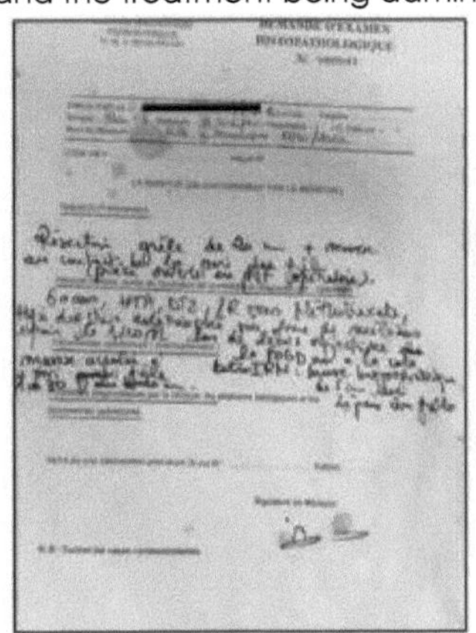
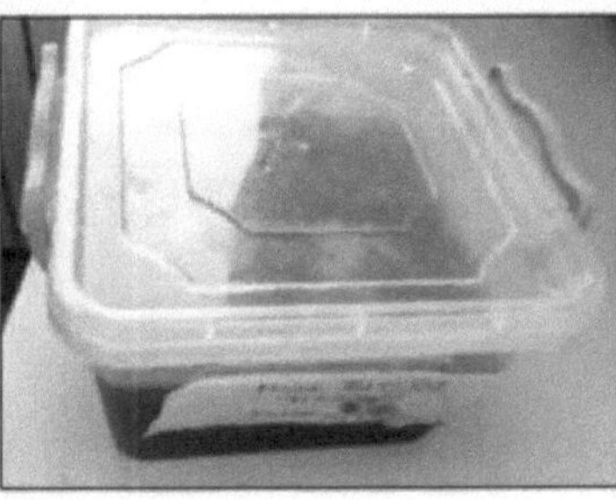

Figure 6: Clinical information sheet accompanying the tumour graft bowel resection specimen

CONCLUSION

Macroscopic examination of grafted intestinal resection specimens contributes to patient management by assessing prognosis and defining important criteria for prescribing any additional post-operative treatment.

REFERENCES

TUBE-DIGESTIF.pdf (uca.ma)
productfile 2047.pdf (facmed-univ-oran.dz)

PART VI

TECHNICAL SHEET: MACROSCOPIC MANAGEMENT OF GASTRECTOMY PARTS

ANATOMY OF THE STOMACH

The stomach is an intra-peritoneal organ located in the left central anterosuperior part of the abdomen.

It follows the resophagus at the level of the cardia and ends at the level of the sphincter of the pylorus, **continuing into the duodenum.**

It is J-shaped, with a small concave upper curve and a large convex lower curve.

It has 4 main regions: the cardia, the fundus, the body and the antrum (antropyloric region).

The **greater epiploon** is attached along the greater curvature.

The **lesser epiploon** lies along the lesser curvature.

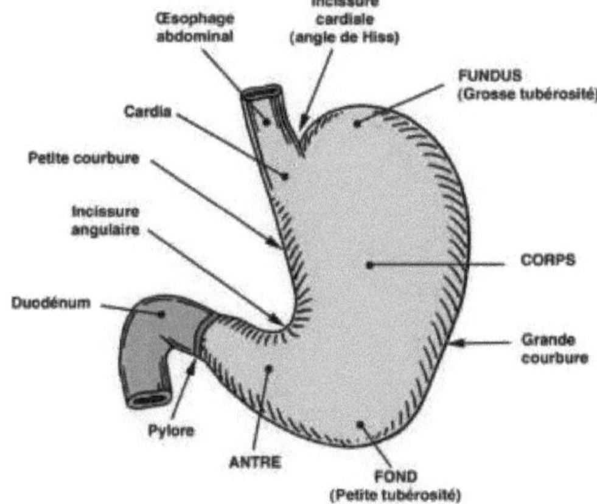

Figure 1: Anatomy of the stomach

Stomach anatomy - General and Digestive Surgery Department at Saint-Antoine Hospital (aphp.fr)

METHODOLOGY

Orientation :

Closed part :

Above: narrower **resophageal tube**

Large convex **curvature**

Large epiploon inserted at the level of the greater curvature

Small concave **curvature**

Small epiploon inserted at the level of the lesser curvature

Bottom: **duodenum**, a tube narrower than the stomach and often longer than the fragment of esophagus.

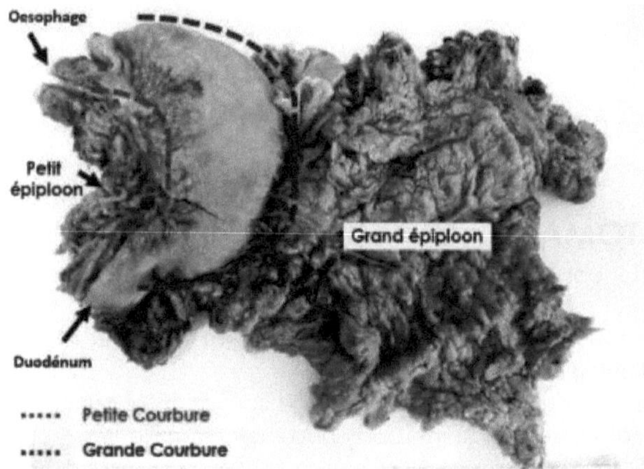

Figure 2: Orientation of a total gastrectomy piece
(Photo of the pathological anatomy department of the CHU Mongi Slim La Marsa)

Weighing and measuring the workpiece :
The gastrectomy part must be weighed
Measurements: use a tape measure to measure the lesser curvature, the greater curvature and the resophageal segment.

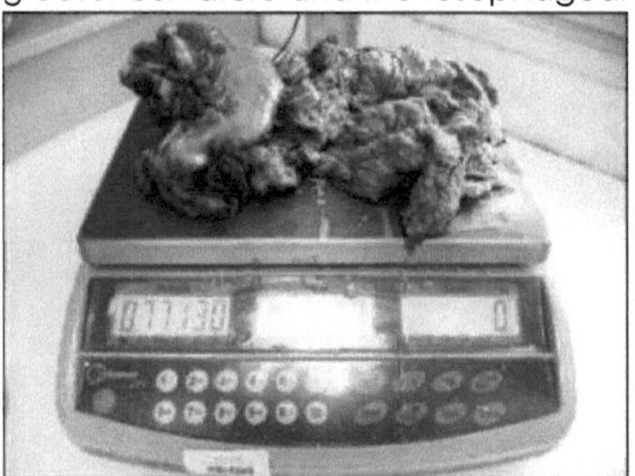

Figure 3: Weighing of a total gastrectomy specimen
(Photo of the pathological anatomy department of the CHU Mongi Slim La Marsa)
Measurement of the Large Curvature Measurement of the Small Curvature

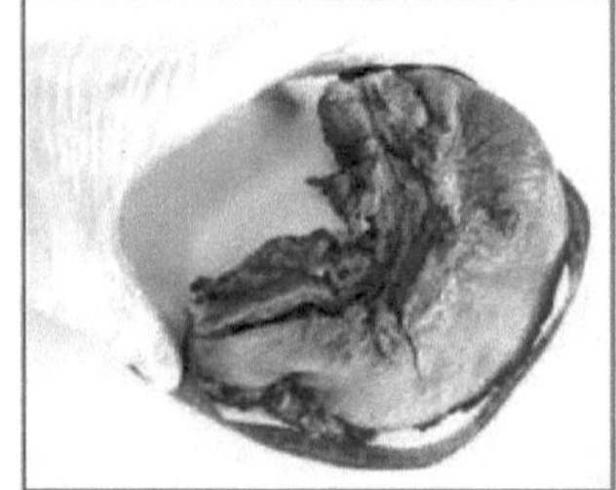
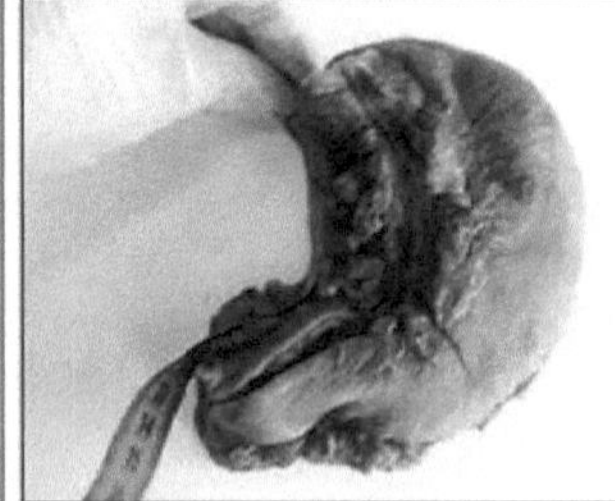

Figure 3 bis: Measurements of a piece of total gastrectomy (Large and Small

36

curvature

curvature)

Opening of the room :

Palpate the piece to locate the tumour area.

Open the section, avoiding cutting the tumour, at best along the large butterfly-wing curvature, otherwise along the small curvature.

Take a photo or possibly a diagram with a legend.

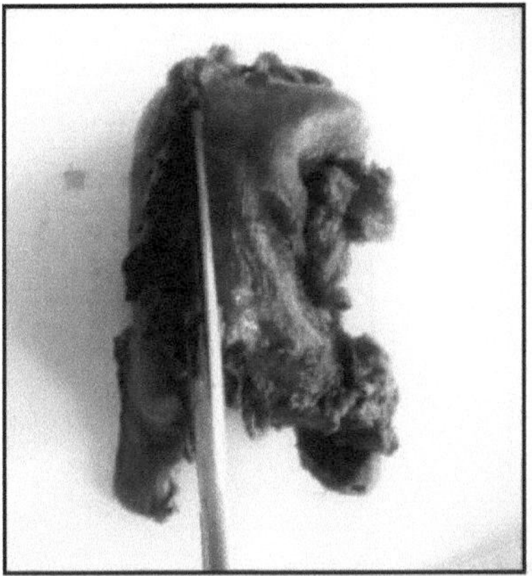
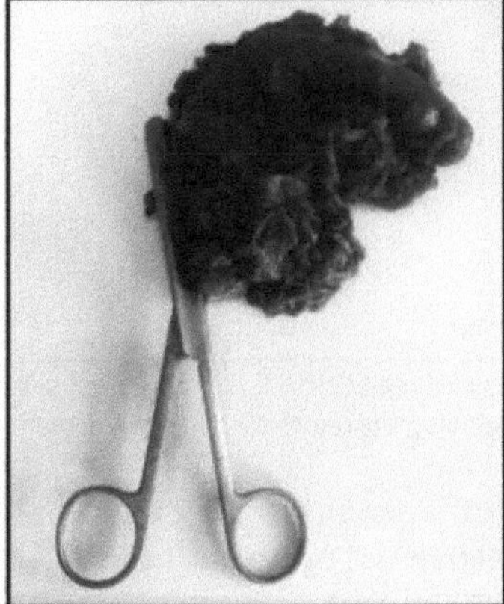

Figure 4: Opening of the total gastrectomy section on the greater curvature using a pair of scissors

(Photo of the pathological anatomy department of the CHU Mongi Slim La Marsa)

External review :

■ Look for an **area of perforation** or **infiltration of the serosa** opposite the tumour area or at a distance, suspected in the presence of

o A frosted appearance of the serosa

o Retraction or even umbilication of the sereuse.

Framing :

The external surface of the cardia if the tumour is reso-cardial (non-peritonealised area to be able to assess the lateral margin)

Any area suspected of peritoneal infiltration;

The limit if infiltration is suspected.

Limit sampling :

The limits are sometimes sent extemporaneously or are sent separately by the surgeon.

If they are full of staples or have not been sent, they will be removed from the operating room.

Always measure the distance between the nearest boundary and the tumour

Total gastrectomy :

■ **If the distance between the tumour and the boundary > 1cm :**

It is sometimes easier to remove the resophageal and duodenal borders from the closed section, but they can also be removed from the open section. Remove the **entire boundary parallel** to the section edge

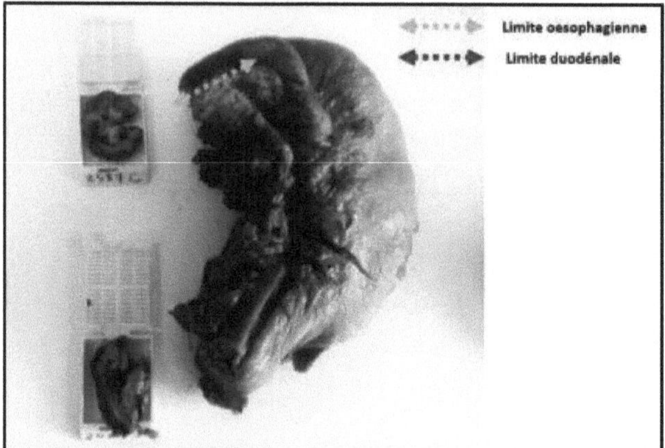

Figure 5: Surgical resection limits on a total gastrectomy specimen
(Photo of the pathological anatomy department of the CHU Mongi Slim La Marsa)

If the distance between the tumour and the boundary is less than 1 cm:
At best, the limits will be taken from the open room.
Take **3 or 4 slices perpendicular** to the boundary (inked boundary)
7. Description of the piece and the tumour :
Description of the piece :
Type of surgery (total gastrectomy, distal gastrectomy, reso-gastrectomy, other)
Length stomach, resophagus, duodenum
Description of the tumour :
Seat, size, appearance
% circumferential invasion
Presence of a perforation
Measurement of extension to the resophagus or duodenum
Distance from nearest boundary
Special case of tumours of the reso-gastric junction :
If EBO (endobrachyresophagus): to be considered as a resophageal tumour.
Otherwise: no consensus definition (tumour considered to be of gastric origin if resophageal invasion **< 2 cm** or **< 50%** or tumour mainly developed on the gastric side, etc.).
Description of neighbouring bodies :
Spleen, transverse colon, liver, diaphragm, pancreas, adrenal glands, kidneys, large intestine, ...
Specify if macroscopic infiltration is evident
Removing the tumour:
0 Make a **series of macroscopic sections (2-3 mm)**

O **Include** at least 3 levels comprising :

s **Maximum infiltration zone**

s The lesion/adjacent **mucosa** ratio

s The ratio of **lesions to resophageal or duodenal mucosa**

s The **lesion/neighbouring organ ratio** if invasion is suspected.

Removal of the mucosa at a distance:

- Systematic sampling of the remote mucosa to look for lesions of gastritis.

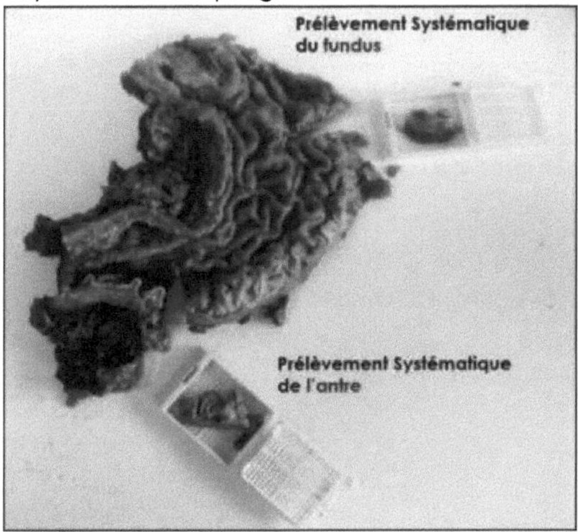

Figure 6 : Systematic removal of the antrum and fundus from a total gastrectomy specimen

(Photo of the pathological anatomy department of the CHU Mongi Slim La Marsa)

Look for associated lesions:

■ **Look for and remove associated lesions (other tumour sites, particularly peritoneal**; ulceration and any mucosal abnormality; small stromal tumour discovered by chance; liponecrosis sites).

Lymph node sampling:

Include all lymph nodes.

If a lymph node is macroscopically tumourous: a slice included in a single block is sufficient.

If not, include the entire lymph node:

At best 1 node per block. It may be necessary to include 1 node.

on several blocks if it is large

There may be several small nodes per block if they are included without being sectioned (specify the number of nodes per block).

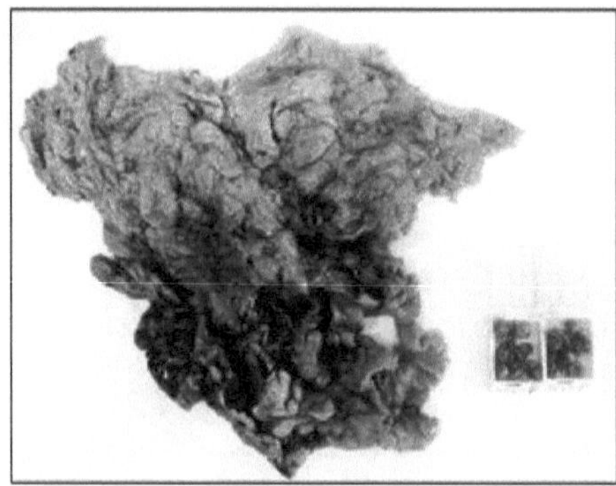

Figure 7: lymph node removal in the greater epiploon
(Photo of the pathological anatomy department of the CHU Mongi Slim La Marsa)

MATERIAL REQUIRED

Fixing agent: The usual fixing agent is 10% buffered formalin.
Scalpel blade - knife
Scissors
Tape measure - Regie plate
Cassettes
Camera

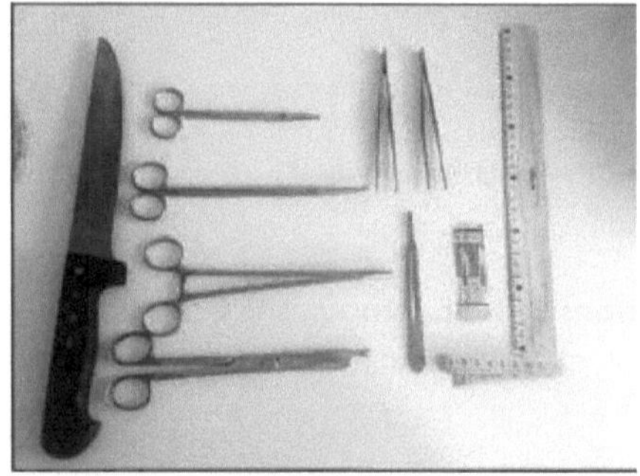

Figure 8: Equipment required for macroscopic management of tumour gastrectomy specimens
(Photo of the pathological anatomy department at CHU Mongi Slim La Marsa)

CONDITIONS AND RULES OF GOOD PRACTICE

The surgical specimen is fixed for 24 - 48 hours in 10% buffered formalin.

Delayed or poor fixation will impair the morphological quality of histological sections. Respect the ratio of tissue volume to fixative volume (1/10).

All gastrectomy specimens must be sent to the pathological anatomy laboratory together with a clinical information sheet describing the history of the disease, the patient's antecedents, the results of the practical paraclinical examinations and the treatment instituted.

40

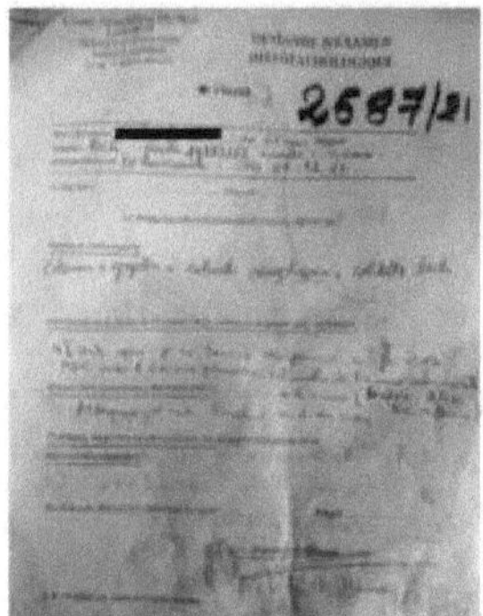

Figure 9: Clinical information sheet accompanying the total gastrectomy specimen to the pathology laboratory
(Photo of the pathological anatomy department of the CHU Mongi Slim La Marsa)

CONCLUSION

■ Macroscopic examination of gastrectomy specimens contributes to patient management by assessing prognosis and defining important criteria for prescribing any additional post-operative treatment.

REFERENCES

productfile 2037.pdf (facmed-univ-oran.dz)

Anatomy of the stomach - General and digestive surgery department, Hopital Saint-Antoine (aphp.fr)

Anatomy of the stomach and resophagus (uca.ma)

PART VII

TECHNICAL SHEET: MACROSCOPIC MANAGEMENT OF A SPLENECTOMY SPECIMEN

INTRODUCTION

Splenic pathology is rare in routine practice compared with lymph node pathology. The main circumstances in which splenectomy occurs are trauma and so-called "encounter" parts following complex abdominal surgery. In most cases, these operations pose no problem, as the splenic parenchyma is only affected by trivial hemorrhagic lesions. However, various pathologies may be responsible for splenomegaly, making analysis of the samples more difficult. This difficulty is due to the existence of a wide range of lesions including tumour pathology (lymphomas, myeloproliferative syndromes, vascular and epithelial tumours), functional disorders and inflammatory diseases.

ANATOMY OF THE SPLEEN

A. General situation

■ **Location**

Intra-peritoneal

Left hypochondrium

Under the diaphragmatic dome

Vascularisation

Arterial: **splenic artery**, branch of the celiac trunk

Venous: **splenic vein**, branch of the portal vein

B. External anatomy

The spleen is shaped like **an irregular tetrahedron** and has :

■ **2 sides :**

External surface **(diaphragmatic)**: convex and smooth, against the diaphragmatic dome

Inner surface **(hilar)**: relatively flat, with a central part

the **splenic hilum**

2 edges :

Front edge: crenele

Back edge: vertical, foamed and rounded

2 poles :

Top pole

Lower pole **(base)**: flattened, triangular, called the colonic facet

C. Macroscopic appearance

Average spleen weight

In children: 17 g

Adults: 200 to 250g

Dark red

Firm consistency

Covered by **a thin, dense, essentially fibro-elastic CAPSULE.**

From this capsule, connective veins are formed which extend into the parenchyma. Cutting :

o **White pulp:** formed by small, whitish nodules, disseminated, measuring 0.5 to 1 mm

o **Red pulp:** reddish tissue surrounding the white pulp

METHODOLOGY

A. Orientation criteria:

Outer surface (diaphragmatic) convex and smooth

Inner side (hilar)

- Notched **front edge**

Prelevement a l'etat frais :

NB: In the event of **suspected malignant haemopathy,** the splenectomy specimen **must be sent fresh,** immediately after exeresis.

Samples for tumour bank

If **malignant haemopathy is suspected, several samples (at least 2 tubes) should be taken for freezing and impressions (Superfrost® slides) should be taken** from the :

Lesion zones in the splenic parenchyma

At least one lymph node in the splenic hilum (at best the largest)

If the sample cannot be frozen, it can be preserved in *RNAlater®* (nucleic acid preservative) and sent to the Regional Reference Tumour Library.

Microbiological sampling

∧ **In the event of infectious pathology,** a fresh sample will be sent to the bacteriology laboratory.

Electron microscopy samples

∧ **If overload disease is suspected,** a fresh sample will be preserved in glutaraldehyde for electron microscopy.

External examination:

- Weigh **and measure the spleen**

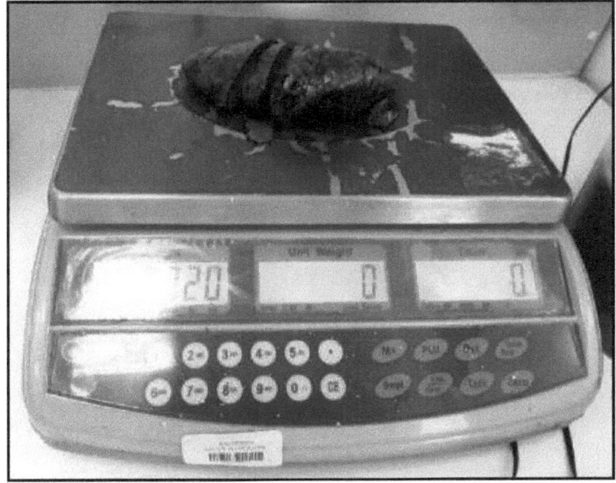

Figure 1: Weighing the splenectomy specimen

■ **Examination of the capsule**

Λ **Particularly in cases of traumatic spleen**

Checking the integrity of the capsule

Look for **subcapsular hematoma**

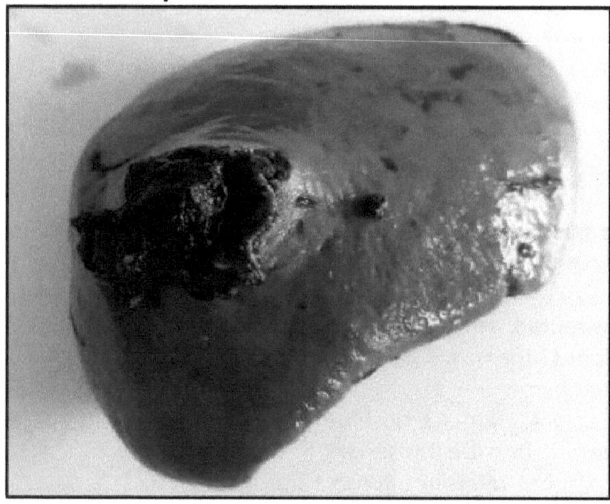

Figure 2: Macroscopic appearance of a capsular rupture of the spleen

Analysis of the splenic hilum :

Search for **ADENOPATHIES :**

Within the fat of the hilum **(particularly in the case of malignant lymphoid pathology).**

Which will be collected **in full.**

Macroscopic sections :

■ **The cuts made MUST BE FINE :**

For **better fixing**

For **optimum morphological analysis**

The slices **are perpendicular to the long axis of the spleen**

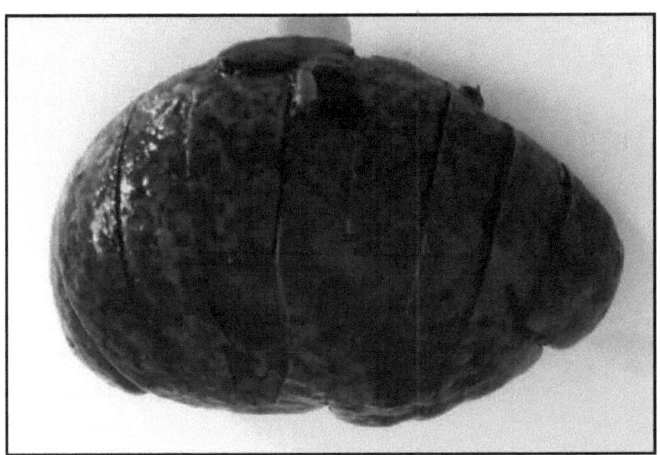

Figure 3: Macroscopic sections of the splenectomy specimen.

F. Mounting

Given the abundance of material available, **all samples (tumour library, imprints, fixation) can be taken.**

NB: It is ESSENTIAL to collect several fragments in 10% buffered formalin (immunohistochemical quality, molecular biology).

G. Description of the room, photographs

Examination and samples will be directed according to the clinical information which is ESSENTIAL

Depending on the clinical context

■ **Traumatic context**: Search and **description**:

Capsular lesions (fracture, subcapsular hematoma)

Parenchymal lesions (number, location)

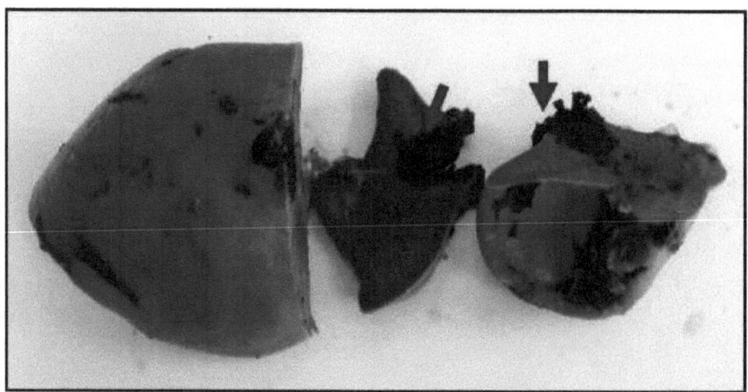

Figure 4: Subcapsular hematoma of the spleen (arrows) (Traumatic spleen)

■ **In the cqse of malignant haemopathy**
- Search for :
Expansion of the white pulp: **= presence of numerous nodules disseminated, whitish, of variable size on a purple background**
- Please specify:
The homogeneous or non-homogeneous nature of the expansion
The size of the largest nodules if expansion is heterogeneous
The presence or absence of foci of necrosis.
expansion of the red pulp: **= red, homogeneous appearance of the parenchyma**

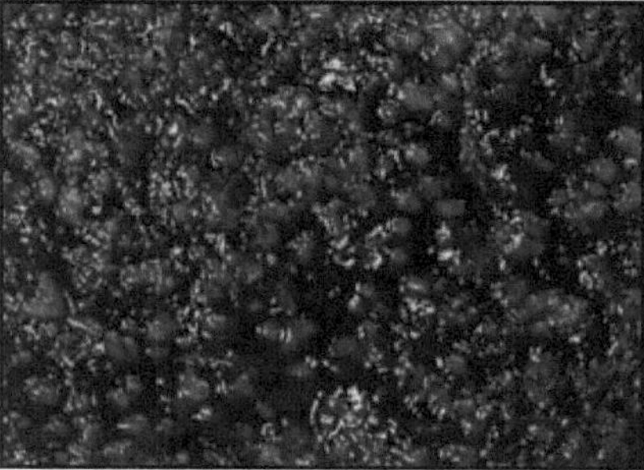

White pulp expansion in splenic marginal zone lymphoma
marginal zone lymphoma

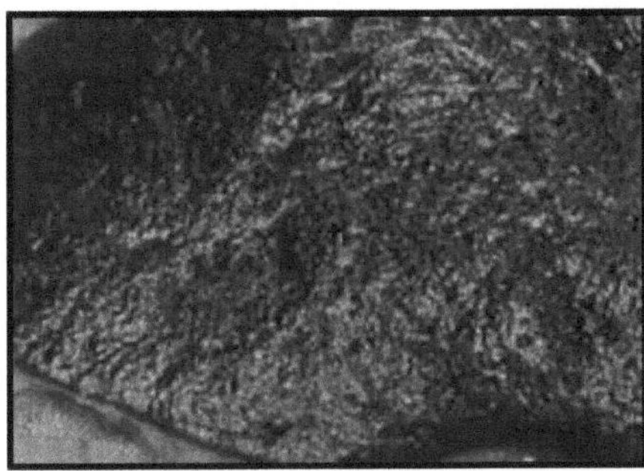

Red pulp expansion in T-cell lymphoma

Non-hematological lesions

∧ Specify :

Appearance of the lesion (colour, contours)

Size

Relationship with the hilum and capsule

H. Taking samples on cassettes. Which one to choose?

■ **In the event of trauma** and in the absence of any suspicious macroscopic lesion

3 or 4 tiered slices

Including 1 slice involving an area of intra-parenchymal hemorrhage

And 1 slice in the transitional zone (pathological spleen / healthy spleen)

■ **In the case of malignant haemopathy**

- If the **white pulp** expands

■ **Homogeneous expansion** :

At least 5 levels on tumour nodules

Including at least two showing the relationship with the capsule

Heterogeneous expansion :

Several levels with priority given to the largest nodules or reworked nodules

2 levels on nodules of homogeneous appearance

∧ If the **red pulp** expands

A minimum of 5 floor levels

Non-hematological lesions

Several levels of lesion

A level showing the relationship with the capsule

At least one level in the transitional zone

A level in a macroscopically healthy zone

No macroscopic lesions

3 or 4 stepped slices, including 1 involving the splenic capsule

In the event of infectious pathology: a fresh sample will be sent to the bacteriology laboratory.

If overload disease is suspected: a fresh sample will be preserved in glutaraldehyde for electron microscopy.

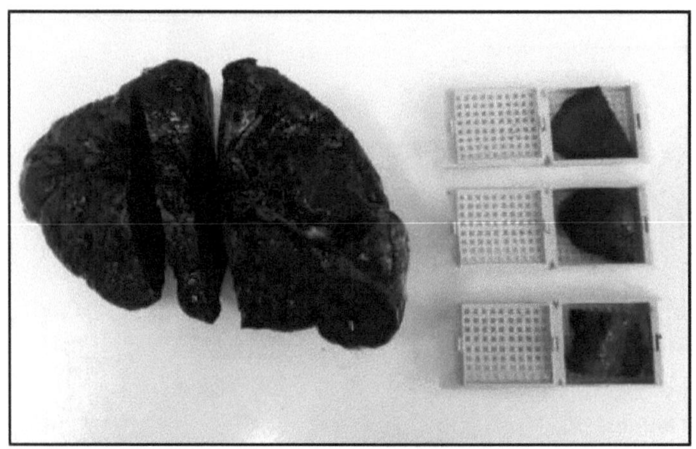

Figure 7 : Samples taken from a fixed splenectomy specimen are placed in cassettes

What to describe

■ **The splenic capsule**

Clarifying your integrity

Look for subcapsular hematoma

■ **The splenic hilum**

Hemorrhagic infiltration (in case of traumatic spleen)

Presence of lymph nodes (number, size)

■ **Splenic parenchyma**

∧ **White pulp**

In the event of expansion of the white pulp, specify :

Whether or not it is homogeneous

Size of the largest nodules

Red pulp

Description of macroscopic lesions

Hematoma (in case of traumatic spleen): number, size

Tumour lesion: size, number, relationship with capsule and hilum

MATERIAL REQUIRED

Fixing agent: The usual fixing agent is 10% buffered formalin.

Scalpel blade - knife

Scissors

Tape measure - Regie plate

Cassettes

Camera

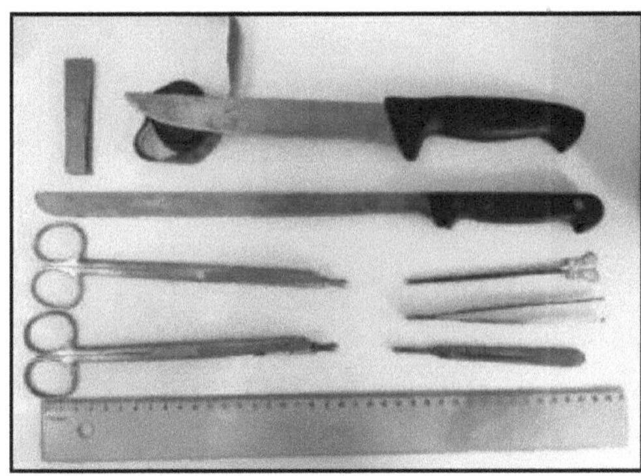

Figure 8: Equipment required for macroscopic examination

CONDITIONS AND RULES OF GOOD PRACTICE

The surgical specimen is fixed for 24 - 48 hours in 10% buffered formalin.

Delayed or poor fixation will impair the morphological quality of histological sections. Respect the ratio of tissue volume to fixative volume (1/10).

All splenectomy specimens must be sent to the pathological anatomy laboratory together with a clinical information sheet detailing the history of the disease, the patient's antecedents, the results of practical paraclinical examinations and the treatment instituted.

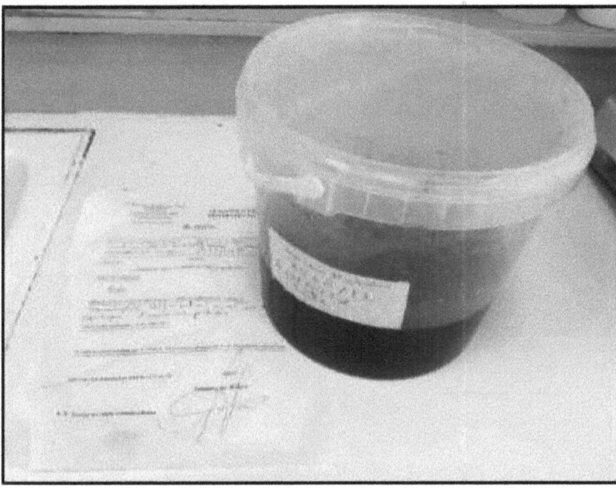

Figure 9: Clinical information sheet accompanying the splenectomy piece

EXAMPLES OF SPLENECTOMY PARTS

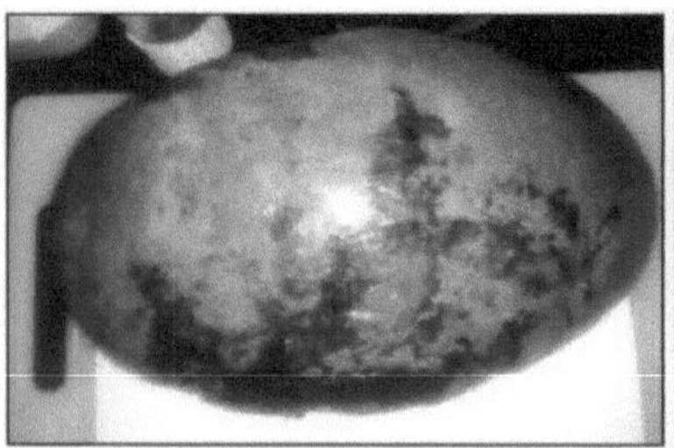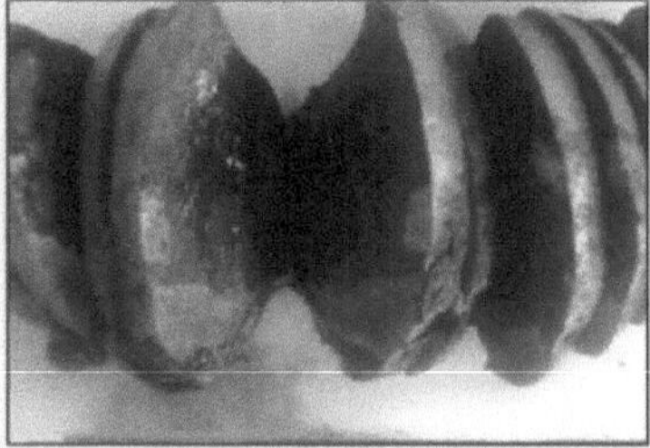

Figure 10: Splenectomy specimen: Mantle cell lymphoma

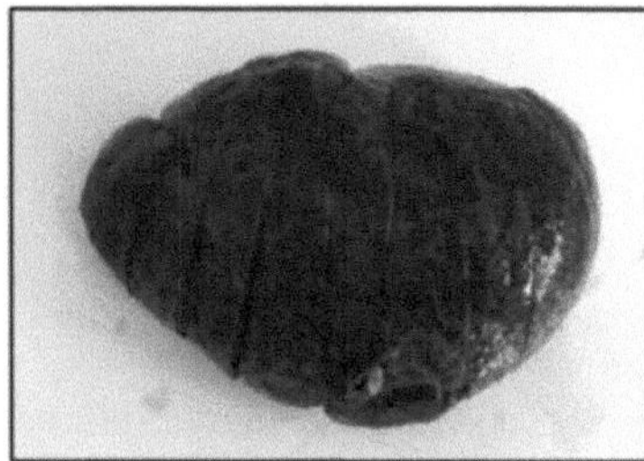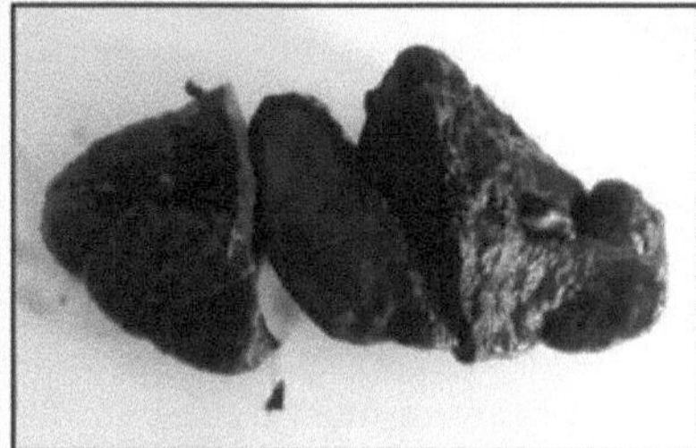

Figure 11: Splenectomy specimen: Idiopathic thrombocytopenic purpura

<u>CONCLUSION</u>

Macroscopic examination of splenectomy specimens contributes to patient management.

Macroscopic examination of splenectomy specimens must be methodical and meticulous.

Adequate sampling of the workpiece is essential if a definite diagnosis is to be made.

<u>REFERENCES</u>

la-rate-cours.pdf (uca.ma) rate.texte (anat-jg.com) Spleen: Anatomy, location and functions | Kenhub

TECHNICAL SHEET: MACROSCOPIC EXAMINATION OF A CEPHALIC DUODENOPANCREATECTOMY SPECIMEN ANATOMY OF THE PANCREAS - GENERAL INFORMATION

Anatomical reminder of the pancreas :

The pancreas is a deep organ located retroperitoneally in front of the large vessels, and extends along an oblique axis upwards and to the left towards the splenic hilum. Concave towards the rear, it wraps around the spine between the 12eme thoracic vertebra and the 3eme lumbar vertebra.

The pancreas is classically segmented into **4 parts**: the feast, the isthmus, the body and the tail.

The head, the widest part, is located inside the duodenal frame. It is

It is bounded at the top by the elements of the hepatic pedicle, on the right by the duodenum and on the left by the mesenteric vessels. The hook *(or uncinatus process, or Winslow's small pancreas)* is an extension of the head at its lower part along the 3rd duodenum. It passes behind the mesenteric vessels and the root of the mesentery.

The isthmus separates the head from the body. It lies anterior to the mesenteric venous axis and projects slightly to the right of the median line. It is separated from the head by a straight line passing through the right edge of the superior mesenteric vein (SMV) to the rear and the axis of the gastroduodenal artery to the front. A parallel straight line passing through the left edge of the VMS separates it from the body.

The body slopes upwards, to the left and backwards. Flattened anteroposteriorly, it follows the concavity of the spine.

The tail continues in the direction of the body after the splenic artery crosses the upper edge of the gland.

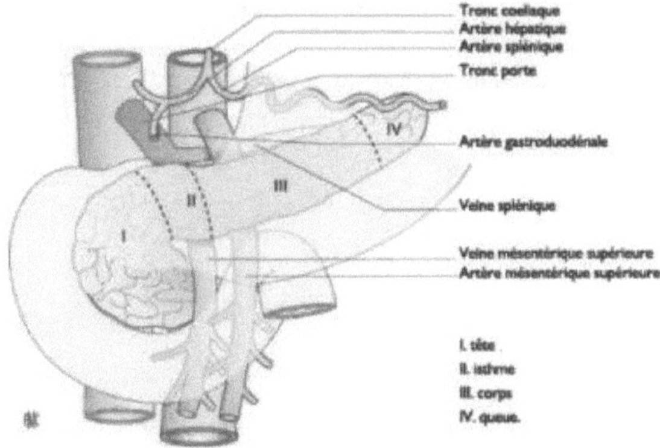

Figure 1: Segmentation of the pancreas ANATOMY AND RADIOANATOMY OF THE PANCREAS (univ-tours.fr)

Cephalic duodeno-pancreatectomy (CPP): or Whipple procedure

+- Takes :
the pancreas with the choledochus (common bile duct) and the gallbladder with the inferior biliary convergence. The latter 2 are sometimes treated separately.
the duodenum and sometimes the distal part of the stomach upstream
-Indications: lesions of the head of the pancreas, choledochus, ampulla of Vater or duodenum.

METHODOLOGY

Weighing the workpiece

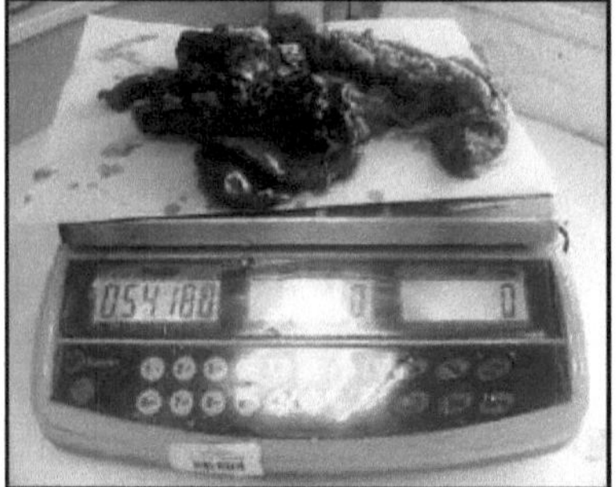

Figure 2: Weighing the cephalic duodenopancreatectomy specimen

Orientation :
Locating and measuring :
Tube :
∧ **Top:** proximal duodenal segment often *short*, sometimes with a recognisable wider gastric segment ∧ **Bottom:** distal duodenal segment often *longer*
Head of the pancreas with the uncus at the bottom, more or less developed
Choledocholith: tube about 1 cm in diameter, behind the head of the pancreas, often bound and identifiable by its yellow-green colour (bile).
The pancreatic border is often superior and anterior. Wirsung's duct may be helpful if it is dilated, otherwise it is hardly visible (its normal calibre is +/- 2 mm).
Retroperitoneal blade: short or long, only correctly identifiable if marked surgically.

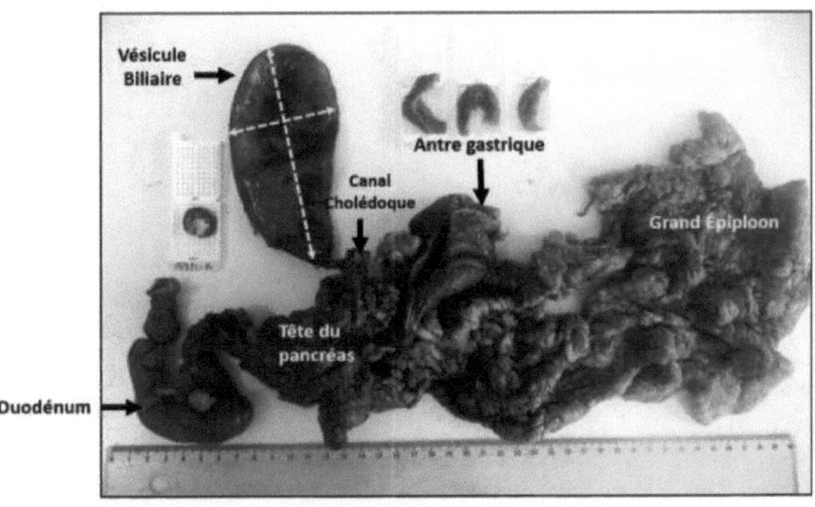

Figure 3: Orientation of the cephalic duodenopancreatectomy section

Setting limits :

Before opening the operating room, **remove the limits of the resections**:
Choledocienne
Pancreatic (often called "isthmic")
Retroperitoneal (only possible if correctly identified surgically)
Lower duodenal
Gastric or upper duodenal

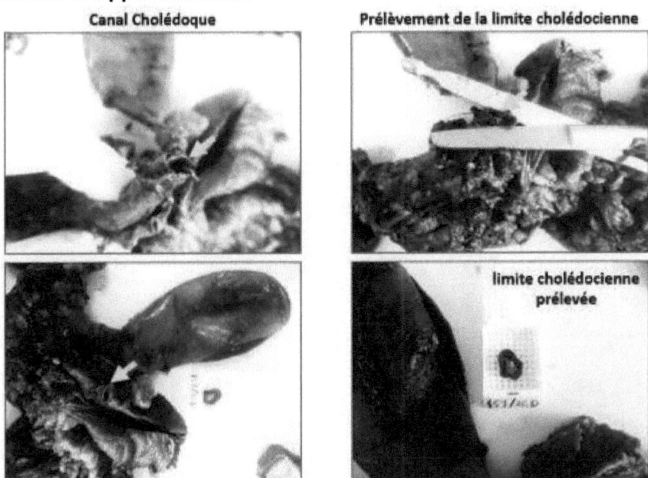

Figure 4: sampling of the Choledocian boundary

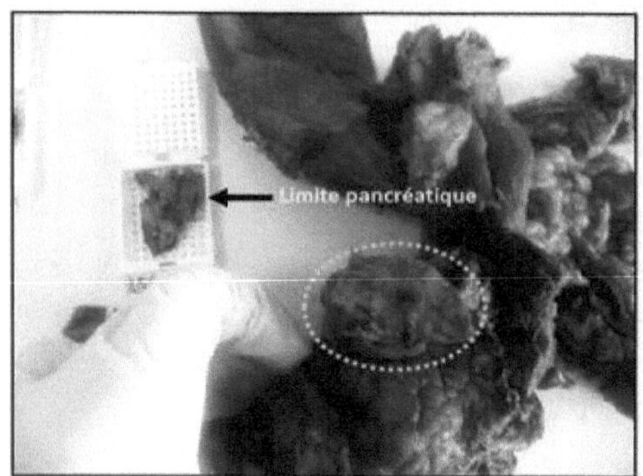

Figure 5: removal of the pancreatic border

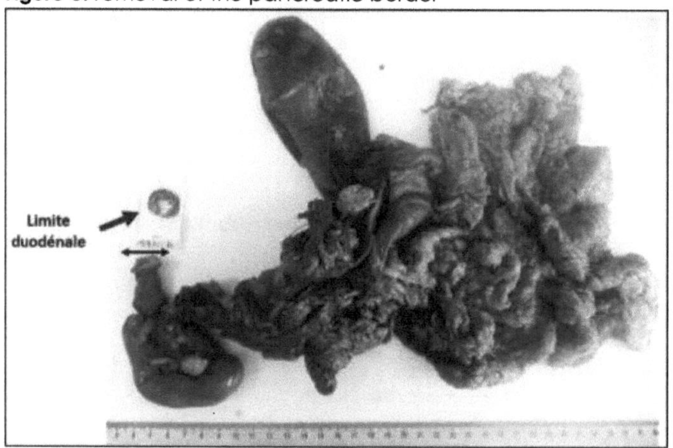

Figure 6: sampling the duodenal border

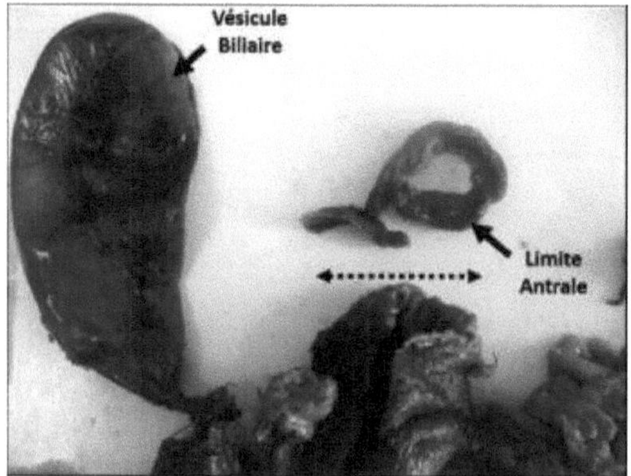

Figure 7: sampling of the gastric antral margin

Particularities of the retroperitoneal boundary :

4 **Retroperitoneal blade (LRP) :**

Cellular-adipose tissue, rich in lymphatics and lymph nodes
Located between the pancreas and the aorta, behind the superior mesenteric vessels,
It can only be sampled correctly if it is identified by the surgeon.
Synonyms: retroporte lamina, posterior pancreatic lamina, retrovascular pancreatic border.

+- Short PRL
If cut flush with the pancreas,
Make 1 LRP block which is both the boundary and the entire retroporte blade

+- Long PRL :
If dissected all the way to the aorta,
To be cut into parallel, marked slices and included *in toto*
The outermost slice is the (upper) boundary *Here block LRP 1*

Framing :
■ In general, it is not necessary to ink this type of part. However, the markings used by the surgeons (Indian ink, surgical sutures, etc.) must be made explicit by the surgeons and are extremely useful for orienting and identifying the limits.

Remove all lymph nodes:
+- To achieve reliable classification, **all lymph nodes must be included and analysed** in their entirety.
4 Optimal regional lymph node dissection usually involves at least 10 nodes for PCD. However, if, *after a thorough search*, no lymph node is metastatic, even if this number is not reached, the tumour will be classified as N0 and not pNx.
+- *The designation pNx is only appropriate if there is no lymph node rësëquë or examined.*
+ At best, "peel" the pancreas: Peeling away the fatty tissue with claw forceps and a scalpel makes it much easier to find the lymph nodes by palpation.
ffi Possibly, in a more traditional way, look for lymph nodes at the end of the macroscopic examination, when the specimen has been completely sliced.

Open and analyse the tube:
Open the tube longitudinally on the anti-pancreatic side, avoiding the papilla.
Examine the entire mucosa for lesions (accessory ampulla, heterotopic pancreas, ulceration by an underlying tumour, etc.), and above all **locate the ampulla, a** small nipple sometimes hidden between mucosal folds.

Opening the pancreas:
+- Open the head of the pancreas
At best, using catheters slid into the choledoch and Wirsung (gun barrel opening).
To see how the lesion relates to the ducts, ampulla and duodenum
Catheterisation is often easier from the limits of the pancreas and choledochus,
But you can also try it from the bulb.
Sometimes the **canals are difficult or impossible to catheterise** (canal orifices difficult to find, deformed canals, stenosis, or even destroyed by a tumour).
S If the 2 channels cannot be catheterised:
First draw the line
■ Then section the pancreas in horizontal parallel cuts to still have relationships with the choledochus, duodenum and ampulla.

Describe the lesion:

Size: at least 2 axes

Aspect

Cystic: unilocular, multilocular? contents: serous, mucous, bloody? developed from or at a distance from the ducts? smooth wall or vegetations? fleshy, infiltrating zone?

Full : well limited / starred

Relations with structures

Wirsung

Choledoque

Bulb

Duodenum

Relationships with limits

Distance between tumour and pancreatic border, taking into account the thickness of the pancreatic cut already isolated.

Description of the peri-tumoral pancreas:

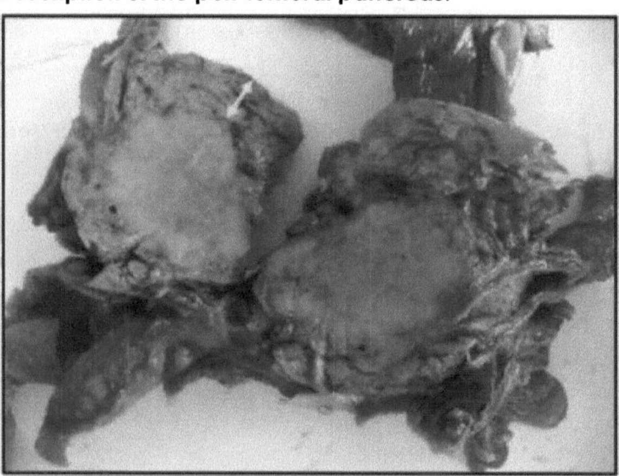

Figure 8: Distance between tumour and pancreatic border (Yellow arrow)

Removing the tumour:

+- Debride the tumour in macroscopically serial slices of 3 mm, perpendicular to the axis of the Wirsung.

4 **Select at least 3 levels of tumour**, taking samples in particular:

Areas of maximum infiltration (ampulla, duodenum, peri-pancreatic adipose tissue)

The tumour/non-tumour junction

Relationships with channels

■ **Ideally, you should also take :**

A level of non-tumourous pancreas, if possible with ducts

The ampoule: at best, sample *tangentially* to the channels *(here block A)*

X **If there is no clearly identifiable tumour** (after neoadjuvant treatment or tumour associated with pancreatitis, for example):

- Or include the entire lesional pancreas.

Either take at least 5 levels in 1er and then, if examination of these 1ers levels shows no obvious tumour, include the reserve.

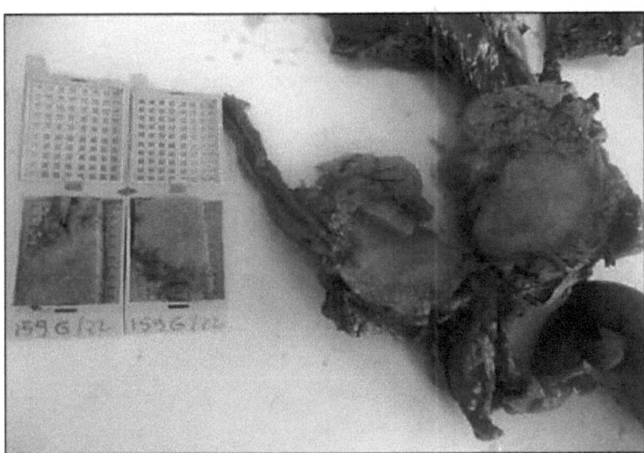

Figure 9: removal of the tumour

Describe and remove associated lesions:
+- Carefully examine the **gastro-duodenal mucosa** to look for and remove any **associated lesions**.
˙˙ Careful examination of the **pancreas** to look for and remove any **associated lesions**
Й Describe the non-tumourous pancreas cut into 3 mm slices (normal / pancreatitis?) and **remove at least one block**.

MATERIAL REQUIRED

Fixing agent: The usual fixing agent is 10% buffered formalin.
Scalpel blade - knife
Scissors
Tape measure - Regie plate
Cassettes
Camera

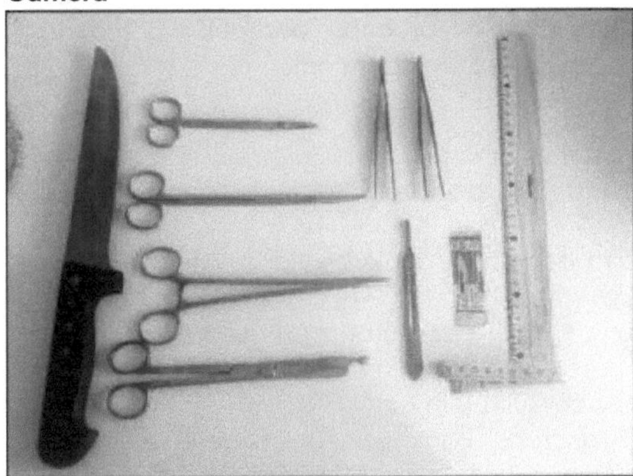

Figure 10: Equipment required for macroscopic processing of cephalic duodeno-pancreatectomy specimens
(Photo of the pathological anatomy department of the CHU Mongi Slim La Marsa)

CONDITIONS AND RULES OF GOOD PRACTICE

The surgical specimen is fixed for 24 - 48 hours in 10% buffered formalin.

Delayed or poor fixation will impair the morphological quality of histological sections. Respect the ratio of tissue volume to fixative volume (1/10).

All cephalic duodeno-pancreatectomy specimens must be sent to the pathological anatomy laboratory together with a clinical information sheet containing the history of the disease, the patient's antecedents, the results of practical paraclinical examinations and the treatment instituted.

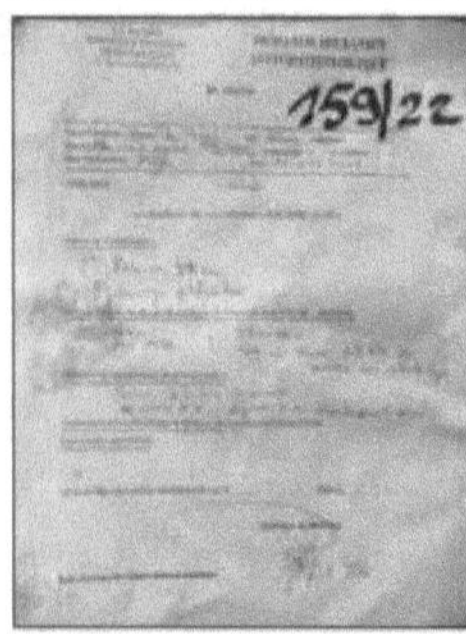

Figure 11: Pathology request form

Importance of surgical information :

Orientation is often difficult because of loss of anatomical relationships and deformity due to fixation, tumour, associated lesions (pancreatitis), etc.

To pinpoint the exact location of the limits, insist that all pancreatic resections are accompanied by a diagram or, better still, explicit markers (ink, thread, staples), particularly at the pancreatic, choledochondral and retro-peritoneal limits.

CONCLUSION

Macroscopic examination of cephalic duodeno-pancreatectomy specimens contributes to patient management by assessing prognosis and defining important criteria for prescribing any additional post-operative treatment.

REFERENCES

Anatomical and physiological bases of the pancreas. Louis Buscail, Barbara Bournet, Nicolas Carrere, Fabrice Muscari and Philippe Otal. Traite de pancreatologie, Chapter 1, 1-21.

Cephalic duodenopancreatectomy - Department of General and Digestive Surgery, Hopital Saint-Antoine (aphp.fr).

Cephalic duodenopancreatectomy | Centre hepato-biliaire Paul Brousse (centre-hepato-biliaire.org).

Surgical anatomy of the pancreas - EM consulte (em-consulte.com).

S. Agostini. Radioanatomy of the pancreas. Radiologie et imagerie medicale - abdominale - digestive, 2017-03-01, Volume 35, Numero 1, Pages 1-13.

PART IX

TECHNICAL SHEET: MACROSCOPIC MANAGEMENT OF AN ANTERIOR RECTAL RESECTION SPECIMEN

ANATOMY OF THE RECTUM

+ The rectum comprises 3 segments (or thirds) each 5 cm high:

Lower third or lower rectum: from the pectineal line and entirely subperitoneal.

Middle third or middle rectum: 2/3 of this segment is subperitoneal.

Upper third or rectum: entirely peritoneal.

ffi The **pectineal line** is the undulating line which separates the anal canal from the lower rectum (yellow arrow).

+ The mesorectum: the **mesorectum** is an anatomical and embryological entity. It is defined as the cellulo-fatty tissue surrounding the lateral and posterior surfaces of the rectum. It is bounded circumferentially by the fascia recti, which can be surgically severed from the pelvic parietal fascia using the total mesorectal excision technique described by Heald. The mesorectum contains the perirectal vessels and lymphatics.

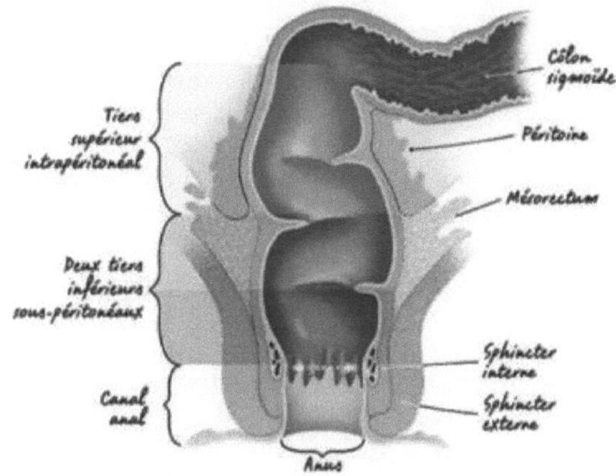

Figure 1: Anatomy of the rectum The rectum - Rectal cancer (e-cancer.fr)

METHODOLOGY

A. Orientation criteria:

1 - Anterior rectal resection specimens with partial exeresis of the mesorectum

- The orientation of the part can be determined by locating the line of reflection of the peritoneum.

Above the line: **upstream** part

Above the line: **downstream** part

+ The line of reflection of the separated peritoneum

The intra-peritoneal portion of the rectum (**upper rectum or recto-sigmoid hinge**)

The subperitoneal portion of the rectum (**middle and lower rectum**)

+- The cul de sac of Douglas is the lowest point of this line, on the **anterior** surface L The portion of **mesorectum** removed extends from the line of peritoneal reflection (pointilles) to the inferior longitudinal limit of the exeresis.

■ **Tumour of the upper rectum** :

The anterior resection only removes part of the mesorectum (this is known as partial mesorectal resection) corresponding to the 5 cm sub-tumour margin recommended for carcinological resection.

2- Anterior rectal resection specimens with total mesorectal exeresis:

- The orientation of the part can be determined by locating the line of reflection of the peritoneum.

Above the line: **upstream** part

Above the line: **downstream** part

4 The line of reflection of the separated peritoneum

The supraperitoneal portion of the rectum (**upper rectum or rectosigmoid hinge**)

The sub-peritoneal portion of the rectum (**middle and lower rectum**)

Followed by the anal canal

+- The cul de sac of Douglas is the lowest point of this line, on the **anterior** surface ∧B

The **pectine line** is the undulating line which separates the anal canal from the lower rectum.

■ **Tumour of the middle and lower rectum** :

+- The anterior resection involves the entire mesorectum (this is known as total exeresis of the mesorectum).

+■ The **mesorectum** extends from the line of reflection of the peritoneum (black dots) to the lower longitudinal limit of the exeresis. The latter may be at the level of the pectin line.

+ In the case of tumours of the lower rectum, the lower part of the exeresis includes a portion of the anal canal (3) and the internal sphincter (inter-sphincter resection).

Abdominoperineal amputation parts :

On the front of the piece, you can see **the line of reflection of the peritoneum**, which separates the two sides of the piece.

The supraperitoneal portion of the rectum (upper rectum or recto-sigmoid hinge)

The sub-peritoneal portion of the rectum (middle and lower rectum),

The anal canal,

And in the distal portion, the anus and perianal region.

B- Measurement, palpation and description of the whole piece and mesorectum

Operating part :

Type of resection

Length of piece

Possible extension of the exeresis to a neighbouring organ (hypogastric plexus, semen vesicle, prostate ...)

Integrity of the mesorectum: Specify whether the mesorectum is complete with a smooth surface or locally incomplete: exposure of the muscularis.

Tumour :

Location (anterior, lateral, posterior)

Dimensions (length, width and circumference)

Distance from the peritoneal reflection line

Distance from **lower longitudinal limit**

Extension to the mesorectum or peritoneum

The tumour can be identified by palpation on a fresh, closed specimen. Certain details can be determined later on an open specimen

C- Opening the part and packaging for optimum hold:

L The specimen must be opened on both sides of the tumour, respecting the 2 cm above and below the tumour, and then washed. This allows the mesorectum opposite the tumour to be respected, which will then be examined and harvested (circumferential margin).

4 Any **associated lesions** (polyp, diverticulum, etc.) are then identified.

4 A **moistened compress** is inserted into the lumen to facilitate tumour fixation.

L The part is **pinned to a rigid support** (in this case a cork plate) and placed under gentle tension before being immersed in the fixative for 48 to 72 hours.

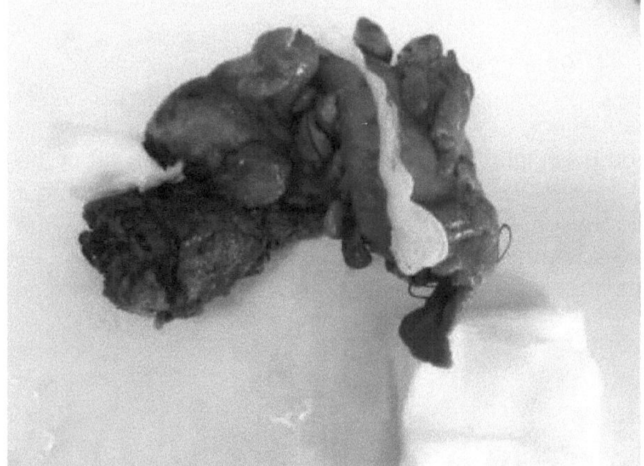

A **moistened compress** is inserted into the lumen to facilitate tumour fixation.

D- Inking of the mesorectum :

After fixation, the surface of the mesorectum or fascia recti is inked. This inking is used to determine the circumferential margin.

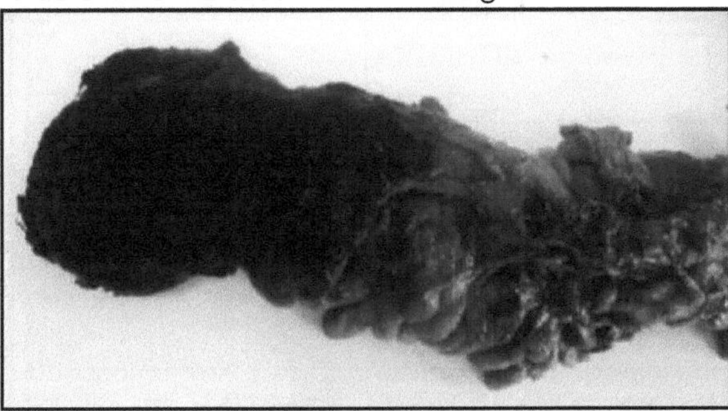

Inking the mesorectum (India ink)

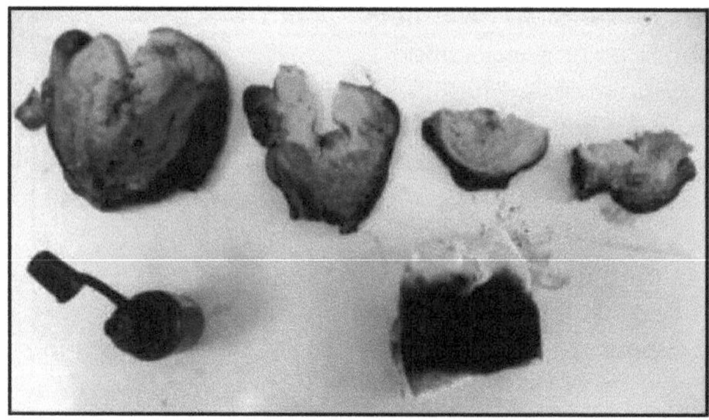

Inking the mesorectum (India ink). The operative piece is then
sliced in series.

E- Macroscopic sections, description :

The unopened peri-tumour zone is cut into macroscopically serrated slices (from the lower end to the upper end) in order to determine the relationship of the tumour directly or of any metastatic lymph nodes to the circumferential margin, the boundary of which has been inked beforehand.

This management also includes analysis of the integrity of the mesorectum in relation to the tumour.

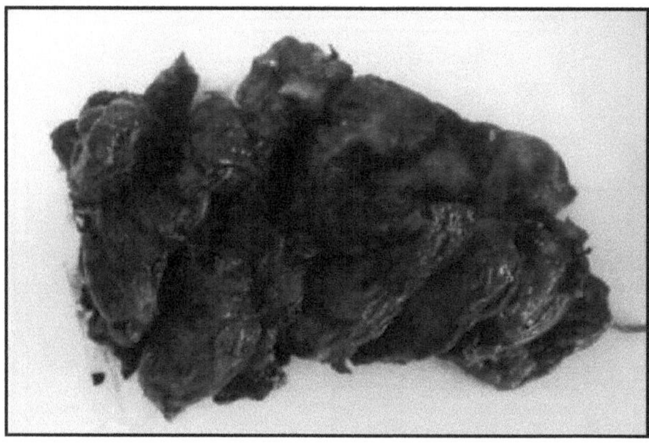

Making macroscopically-serious sections of the workpiece

F- Selection of samples for analysis :

т- **Three to 5 trans-tumour slices** should be taken, giving priority to areas of **maximum** tumour **infiltration** and to those where the **circumferential margin** (distance between the tumour and the recti fascia; arrow) is the narrowest.

+ All nodes must be sampled and individualised (1 node/cassette). Any tumour node or nodule tangent to the recti fascia must be harvested as a single unit. This will allow the value of the circumferential margin to be determined in relation to any tumour node or nodule.

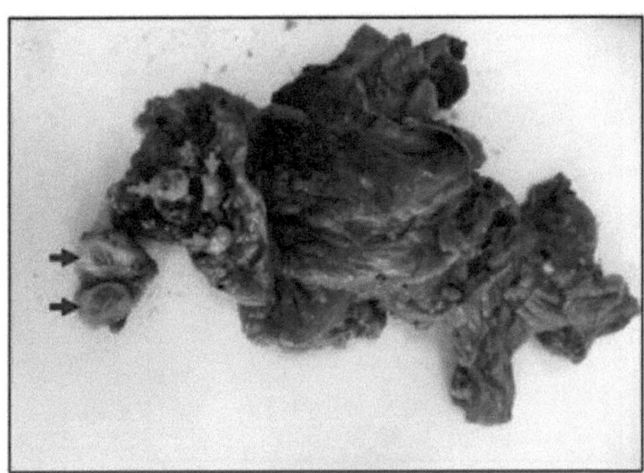
Thorough search for lymph nodes (arrows) by slicing the mesorectum.

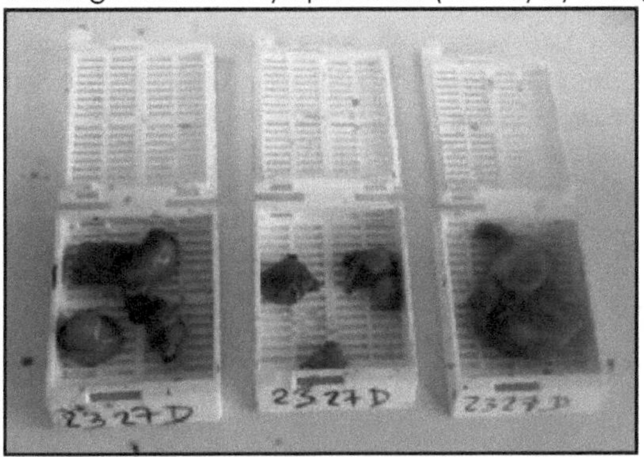

Lymph nodes removed from the mesorectum are
placed in cassettes.
The rest of the specimen must be carefully examined and any **associated lesions** (polyps, diverticula, etc.) removed.

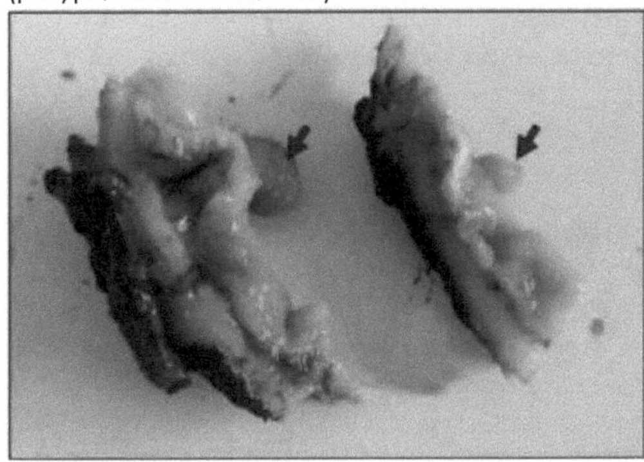
Two polyps (blue arrows) are removed from the operating room
+- The **proximal and distal longitudinal limits**, and the **rectal flange** where appropriate, must be distinct.

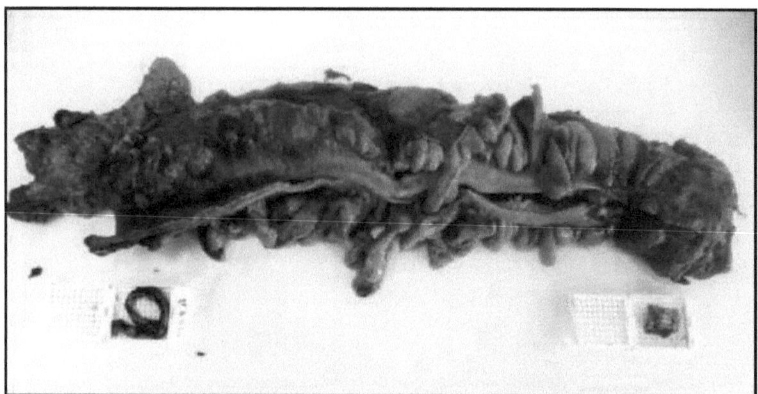

Figure 9 : Proximal and distal longitudinal limit sampling.

+- In the case of a tumour located less than 1 cm from the exeresis border, transtumoural sections **perpendicular to the border** (arrows) are preferable in order to provide the best information on the distal longitudinal margin.

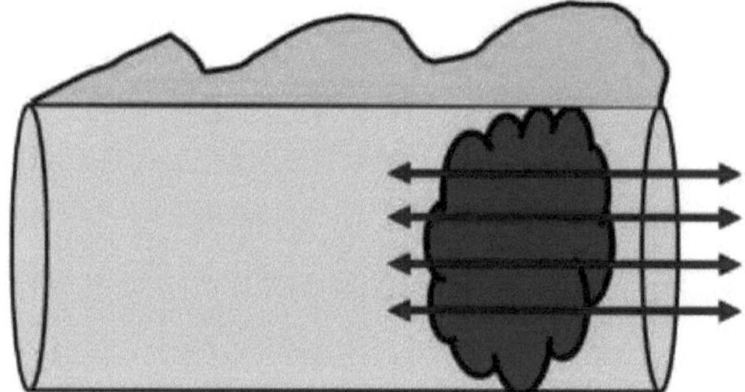

Figure 10: Trans-tumour slices **perpendicular to the boundary** (arrows) are to be preferred in cases where the tumour is less than
preferred in the case of a tumour located **less than 1 cm from the exeresis limit.**

What to collect

Proximal and distal longitudinal **limits**

Tumour :

maximum tumour and lymph node infiltration levels / inked circumferential resection margin

tumour/non-tumour tissue junction (3 to 5 levels of cut)

in the case of a tumour less than 1 cm from the distal longitudinal border: indicate the border on transtumoural sections taken perpendicular to the border

Nodes: meticulous search for all nodes, including all if macroscopically non-tumourous or part if tumourous, 1gg/cassette. If less than 12 or 8 lymph nodes, repeat the section with or without the aid of additional techniques (Bouin's fluid surfixation, fat clearance, etc.).

Any other associated lesion: polyps, diverticula, ulcerations, etc.

MATERIAL REQUIRED

Fixing agent: The usual fixing agent is 10% buffered formalin.
Scalpel blade - knife
Scissors
Tape measure - Regie plate
Cassettes
India ink - Compresses
Camera

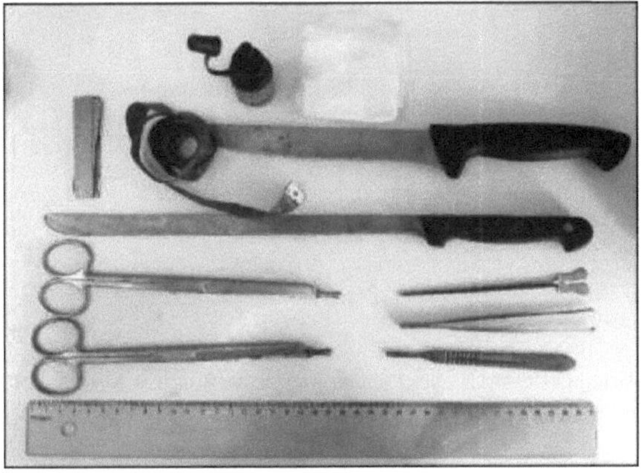

Figure 11: Equipment required for macroscopic processing of anterior resection specimens

CONDITIONS AND RULES OF GOOD PRACTICE

The surgical specimen is fixed for 24 - 48 hours in 10% buffered formalin.

Delayed or poor fixation will impair the morphological quality of histological sections.
Respect the ratio of tissue volume to fixative volume (1/10).

All previous rectal resection specimens must be sent to the pathological anatomy laboratory together with a clinical information sheet describing the history of the disease, the patient's past history, the results of practical paraclinical examinations and the treatment administered.

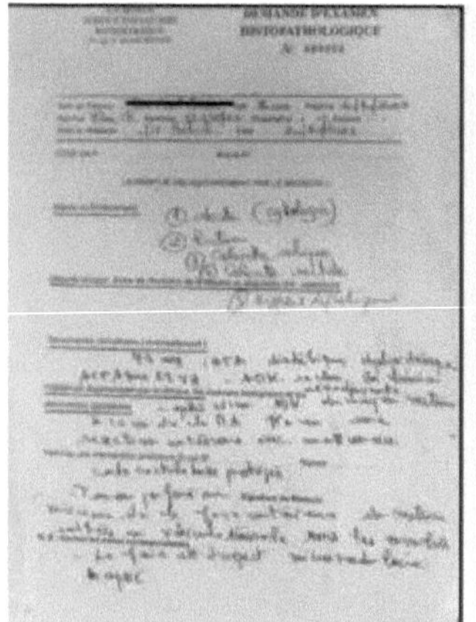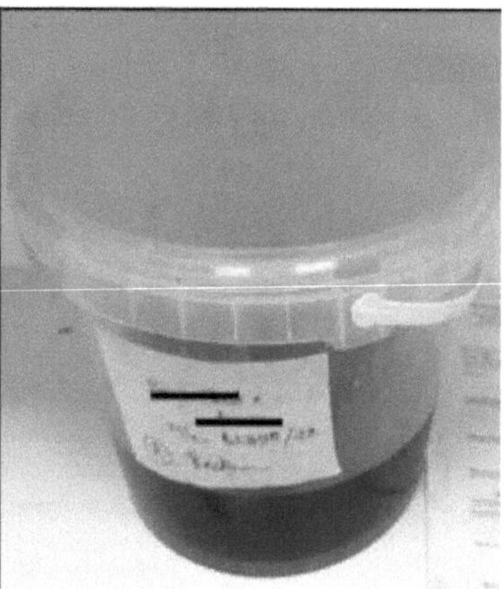

Figure 12: Clinical information sheet (left) accompanying the anterior rectal resection specimen received in a labelled vial containing formalin.

CONCLUSION

■ Macroscopic examination of anterior rectal resection specimens contributes to patient management by assessing prognosis and defining important criteria for prescribing any additional post-operative treatment.

REFERENCES

productfile 2053.pdf (facmed-univ-oran.dz)

RECTUM (univ-batna2.dz)

PART X

TECHNICAL SHEET: MACROSCOPIC MANAGEMENT OF COLORECTAL LIVER METASTASES
METHODOLOGY
Orienting the workpiece:
Locating the Glisson capsule
Section slice (inking optional)
The supra-hepatic veins
The edges of the liver
Ligaments
The vesicular fossa
Size and weight of sample :
Tumorectomies: capsular diameters and depth
Hepatectomies: weight and height according to its 3 axes
Describe :
Packaging : 10% buffered formalin / fresh state
External appearance: split / atrophy / parenchymal dysmorphia / therapeutic embolisation of portal veins / capsular adhesions (peritoneum, neighbouring organ) / abnormal colouring
Pre-slicing for better fixing:
- Slices of 2 - 3 cm, in book leaf (paper), left to set for 24 hours in 10% buffered formalin.
Releasing the fixed part:
Horizontal slices every 5 mm (hepatectomies) or perpendicular to the surface of the liver (subcapsular lumpectomy)
Use the diagram to locate tumours
Check for any areas of the capsule that may have become upturned

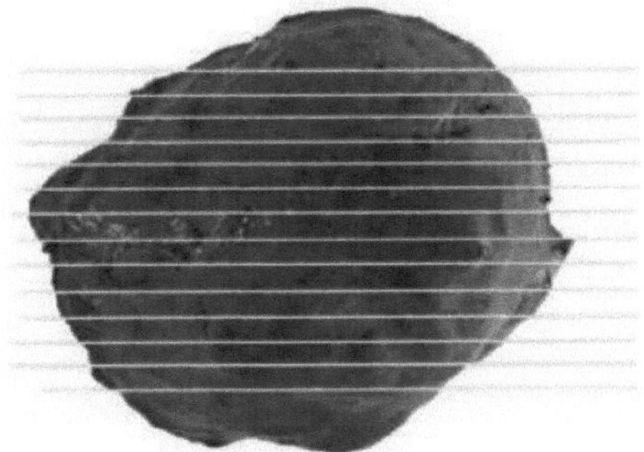

Fig1. Horizontal slices every 5 mm

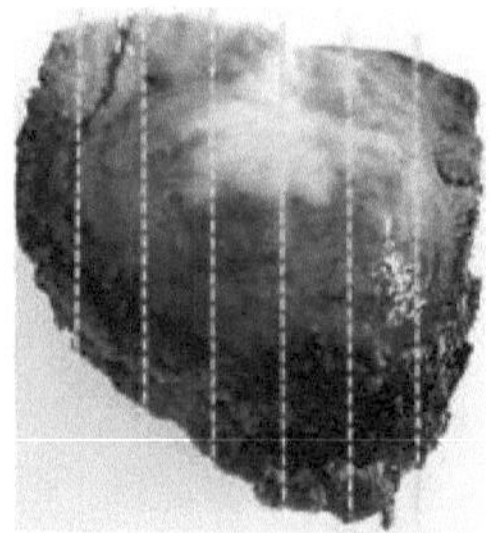

Fig.2: Lumpectomy specimen: perpendicular slices every 5 mm

Photos of tumour slices and photo identification

Describing on a diagram

The number of tumours

Diameters (2 for large tumours, 1 for small tumours); A X B mm

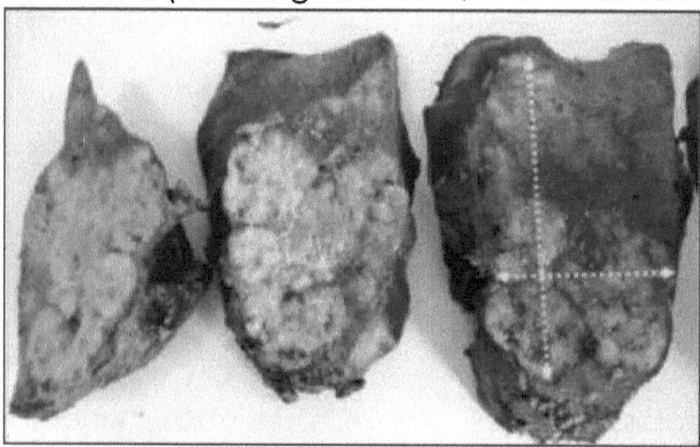

Fig.3 : measuring the two diameters for large tumours

- Minimum healthy margin (L = x mm)

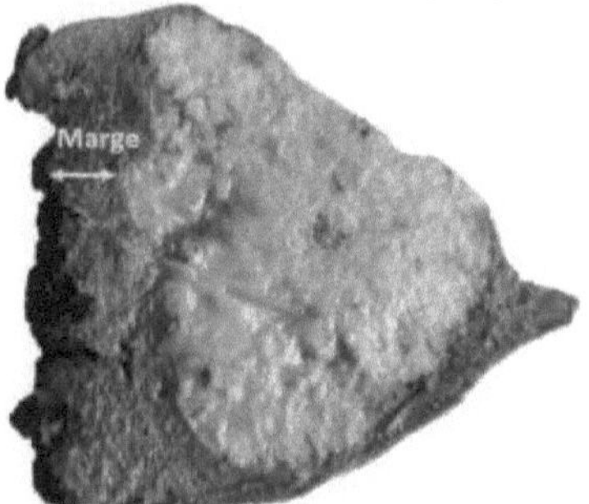

Fig. 4: Surgical margin

Seat (segment ? subcapsular or deep ?)

Specify if mal limit or confluent nodules

Particular appearance? gelatinous, necrosis, calcified

Particular extension: Glisson's capsule, peritoneal adhesion, portal spaces, large vessels, bile ducts

The non-tumorous liver: portal thrombosis, parenchymal congestion, steatosis, atrophy, etc.

Collect and place in cassettes

- Metastases :

1-3 blocks/metastasis, depending on size and heterogeneity

Liver/tumour interface

Tranche showing minimum healthy margin

Peritoneal adhesions

Rupture of the Glisson capsule, emboli

Non-tumourous liver: 1 or 2 blocks

Pedicular ganglion (if present)

MATERIAL REQUIRED

Fixing agent: The usual fixing agent is 10% buffered formalin.

Scalpel blade

Indian ink

Cassettes

Camera

Conclusion

In conclusion, the "Practical Guide to Macroscopy in Pathological Anatomy - Essential Guidelines" is much more than just a manual; it is an indispensable companion in the complex world of surgical specimen analysis. Through precise guidelines and rigorous protocols, this guide lights the way for pathologists, helping them to decipher the mysteries buried in every tissue examined.

Macroscopic examination is an essential starting point, revealing crucial information for the diagnosis, prognosis and treatment of pathological conditions. From meticulous fixation to meticulous inclusion, each stage of this process requires special attention and expert know-how to guarantee reliable, meaningful results.

By embracing the complexity of the tissues examined, navigating the nuances of lesions and interpreting the clues left in each specimen, pathologists continue to be the guardians of diagnostic accuracy and quality of patient care.

Thus, this guide, by virtue of its essential role in the practice of pathological anatomy, remains a fundamental pillar for all those engaged in the quest to understand and solve medical puzzles. Through its diligent and respectful use of established protocols, it contributes tirelessly to the advancement of medical science and to the well-being of patients throughout the world.

Resume

The "Practical Guide to Macroscopy in Pathological Anatomy" is an essential resource for pathologists, offering detailed protocols for the macroscopic examination of various organs such as the appendix, gall bladder, digestive polyps, etc. Each protocol guides professionals through the precise analysis of specimens, from the identification of lesions to the making of key diagnostic decisions. Each protocol guides professionals through the precise analysis of specimens, from identifying lesions to making key diagnostic decisions. By covering a diverse range of organs and lesions, this guide reflects the commitment of pathologists to perfecting their skills in order to provide top-quality care. It represents a crucial pillar in the field of pathological anatomy, contributing to improved diagnosis, treatment and patient outcomes worldwide.

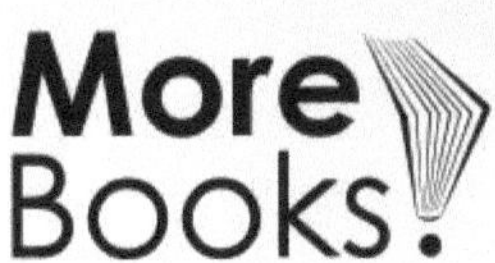

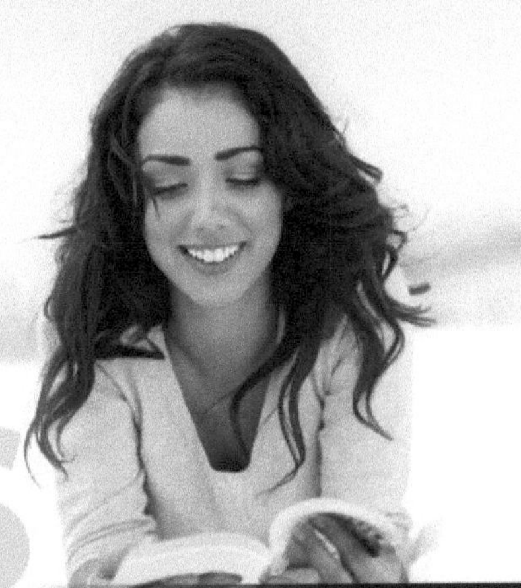

yes
I want morebooks!

Buy your books fast and straightforward online - at one of world's fastest growing online book stores! Environmentally sound due to Print-on-Demand technologies.

Buy your books online at
www.morebooks.shop

Kaufen Sie Ihre Bücher schnell und unkompliziert online – auf einer der am schnellsten wachsenden Buchhandelsplattformen weltweit! Dank Print-On-Demand umwelt- und ressourcenschonend produzi ert.

Bücher schneller online kaufen
www.morebooks.shop

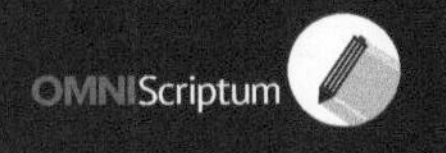

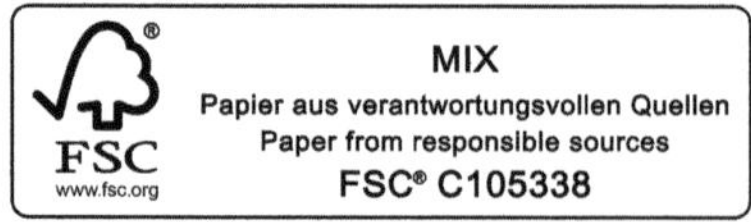

Printed by Books on Demand GmbH, Norderstedt / Germany